Essential Primary Care Computing
A Practice Guide

This book is dedicated to Enn

Essential Primary Care Computing
A Practice Guide

Tony Rennison, BSc, PhD
Specialist Associate Dean – IT/IT Management
Thames Postgraduate Medical and Dental Education
University of London

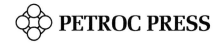

PETROC PRESS

Petroc Press, an imprint of LibraPharm Limited

Distributors

Plymbridge Distributors Limited, Plymbridge House, Estover Road, Plymouth PL6 7PZ, UK

Copyright

©1999 LibraPharm Limited

All rights reserved. No part of this publication may be reproduced, stored in a retrieval system, or transmitted in any form or by any means, electronic, mechanical, photocopying, recording or otherwise, without prior permission from the publishers.

While every attempt has been made to ensure that the information provided in this book is correct at the time of printing, the publisher, its distributors, sponsors and agents make no representation, express or otherwise, with regard to the accuracy of the information contained herein and cannot accept any legal responsibility or liability for any errors or omissions that may have been made or for any loss or damage resulting from the use of the information.

Published in the United Kingdom by
LibraPharm Limited
3b Thames Court
High Street
Goring-on-Thames
READING
Berkshire
RG8 9AQ
UK

A catalogue record for this book is available from the British Library

ISBN 1 900603 66 7

Printed and bound in the United Kingdom by
Alden Press, Osney Mead, Oxford OX2 0EF

Contents

Foreword   *xi*
Preface   *xii*
Acknowledgements   *xiii*

1. Introduction to General Practice Computing   1

Introduction   1
The Benefits of General Practice Computing   2
   The Ease of Routine Administrative Operations   2
   The Ease of Authorised Practice Staff in Accessing Information   2
   Bulk Reporting   3
   The Benefits of Practice Computerisation for Staff, GPs and
      Patients   3
   Benefits to GPs   3
   Benefits to the Practice Team as a Whole for Administration   4
   Benefits to Patients   5
   Telemedicine   6
The History of Primary Care Computing   6
Background to Current Systems   7
Basic Uses of General Practice Computer Systems   9
Advanced Uses of the System   10
Types of Hardware   11
A Brief Guide to the Most Important Features of PCs   13
   The Case   13
   The Keyboard   14
   The Motherboard   14
   The Processor – the CPU   14
   RAM   15
   Cache   16
   Input/Output (I/O) Ports   16
   Hard Disk   16
   Floppy Disks   17
   Video Card   17
   Monitor   17
   Operating Systems   18
   Printers   18
   Other Hardware   19

2. How to Select a General Practice System　21

Assessing Aims　21
Coding Systems　26
　Arbitrary　26
　RCGP　27
　ICD9, ICD10　27
　OXMIS　27
　Read　27
Read Codes　27
Choosing a Shortlist of Computer System Suppliers　29
　Users' Input　29
　Published Reviews　30
　In-practice Knowledge　30
　Local Practices　30
　Dispensing Status　30
　Financial Factors　31
　Clinical or Administrative Systems　31
　Multiple Sites　31
Supplier Demonstrations　32
　Arranging Demonstrations　32
　Taking Charge of the Session　33
Other Methods of Viewing Systems　33
Visits to Exhibitions　33
Visits to Other Practices　34
Borrowing a System　34
Other Considerations　35
Support Record　35
Deciding on a Specification　36
Using Professional Facilitation　37
　Ordering the System　37

3. Planning the Initial Use of the General Practice System　39

Introduction　39
General Points on Implementation　39
　Why?　40
　What?　40
　Who?　40
　Where?　40
　When?　41
　When Should the Practice as a Whole be Introduced to the Use of the System　41
　How Should the Practice as a Whole be Introduced to the Use of the System　42

Strategies and Practical Issues	42
Manual Data Entry	42
Electronic Data Entry	44
Registration Data	44
Prescribing	46
Cytology and Immunisations	49
Simple Predefined Searches	49

4. Further Uses of the General Practice System   53

General Points	53
Recall Letters	54
Patient Information	55
Implementing a Preferred Read Code List	56
Comprehensive Data Entry	58
Major Events Only	59
Selected Health Data Entry Only	59
How Should Clinical Data be Entered?	60
Structured Electronic Records	60
Templates	61
Searches, Audits and Reports	63
Indexes	64
ANDs, ORs and NOTs	65
Read Codes and Searching	65
Export to PCs for Further Processing	66

5. The AAH Meditel System   67

Basic Information	67
Registration	68
Notes	69
Problems and Problem Headings	71
Medication	73
SOPHIE	73
Reporting	75
The Report Generators	76
From Index...	76
Filters	77
Sort Order, Format and Output	78
Recent Changes	79

6. The EMIS System 81

Basic Information 81
Registration 82
Medical Record 83
    Medical Record Mode 83
    Consultation Mode (CM) 84
    'Problems' in EMIS 86
Medication 86
Templates 88
Reporting 89
Patient Searches 90
Audit Searches 91
Recent Developments 92

7. The VAMP Medical System 95

Basic Information 95
Registration 96
Patient Notes 97
    Prevention Screen 97
Medical History 98
Prescribing 99
Freehand 99
Macros 100
Standard Reports/Practice Analysis 101
Report Generator and Freehand Reports 102
Freehand Searches 104

8. Other Systems 107

Introduction 107
VAMP Vision 107
    Registration 108
    Patient Data 108
    Reporting 111
    Conclusions 112
AAH Meditel System 6000 113
    Registration 114
    Patient Data 115
    Reporting 118
    Conclusions 118
The Torex (GP Manager) System (Previously Ambridge) 119
    Registration Data 120

Clinical Data	120
Searches	122
Conclusions	122
The Torex Premier System	123
Registration	123
Patient Data	124
Reporting	126
Conclusions	127
Amsys	128
Registration	128
Patient Data	129
Searches	130
Conclusions	131
Seetec GP Professional	132
Registration Data	133
Patient Data	133
Searches	135
Conclusions	135

9. Communications   139

Introduction	139
Registration Links	139
Items of Service Links	140
Pathology Links	141
Pathology Links – A Practical Example	141
Other Links	142
Email	142
Discharge Letters	144
Hospital Appointments	144
Telemedicine	144
The Internet	145
Hardware and Communications	147
Hardware and the Internet	147
Accessing Practice Systems	148
Portable Computers	149

10. Using PCs in General Practice   151

Introduction	151
Spreadsheets	152
Spreadsheet Development	152
Word Processing	156
Microsoft Word	156

Corel WordPerfect	156
Lotus Word Pro	157
Accounts Software	157
Advantages	157
Disadvantages	157
Other Software	158
Desk-top Publishing	159
Presentation Software	159
Personal Information Managers (PIMs)	159
Distance Learning Material	160
Reference Material	160
Payroll	161
Non-clinical Database Systems	161
Integration with the Clinical System	161

Appendix 1 Glossary of Terms   **165**

Appendix 2 Recommended Minimum Specification for a Server   **167**

Appendix 3 Recommended Minimum Specification for a PC Workstation   **168**

Appendix 4 The Essentials of Virus Protection   **169**

What is a PC Virus?	169
Boot/Partition Sector Virus	169
'Normal' Viruses	169
Windows-specific Viruses	170
Macro Viruses	170
Types of Anti-virus Software	170
Scanners	170
Monitors	171
Prevention – the Adoption of Rules and Procedures	171
Suggested Anti-virus Software	172

Appendix 5 Suppliers Mentioned in the Text   **173**

Appendix 6 Further Reading   **174**

Index   **176**

Foreword

General practice is once again going through a time of rapid change. The establishment of primary care groups has meant that practices will now focus on the quality of care and the efficient use of resources. Furthermore, practices will now be working together in groups to plan and monitor the delivery of clinical care. Practice information requirements will continue to increase, for information that is both accurate and timely. Both the continuing demands facing a practice and the current changes will mean that an efficient and effective computer system will be essential. It will be those practices that have an information technology policy and system that will have an advantage in the future. While many practices are computerised, it is the level to which they are using the computer system that is important. Most practices could further improve their use of information technology.

This book aims to help both practices that may be considering acquiring a computer system for the first time and those that already have a computer system. For those with a system, this book will help them either to maximise their current use of it, or to change to another system. It starts by looking at the benefits of a computer system to the practice and then takes the reader through the significant stage of selecting a system to match the practice's information technology requirements. The reader is then taken through the difficult implementation phase. Since communication with other parts of the Health Service is becoming a core function, this is also considered here in some detail.

Tony Rennison has considerable expertise in primary care computing. He has spent a number of years working with practices to help them develop their information technology requirements. His audit courses, held within the practice, have helped many to improve the use of their computer systems. Hence he has an unusual in-depth knowledge of most of the leading primary-care computer systems. This is evident in the book, with chapters on all of the main computer systems that are even up-to-date with the latest emerging Windows versions.

This book covers most aspects of primary care computing and will be valuable both to those looking for their first system and to those wanting either to improve or change their current system.

Dr Peter Orton, FRCGP, MMedSci
Senior Lecturer
Institute of General Practice
University of Exeter

Preface

I have been working in the field of general practice computing for many years now. My background is not in primary care but in pure science with a strong computing bias.

Most of my day-to-day work is practice based – organising courses with GPs and other members of the practice teams so as to develop the use of the clinical computer system and personal computers (PCs) in the practice.

Many of the problems encountered are repeated in practice after practice, and for this very reason I have written this book. It is not intended to be a comprehensive review of the theory of practice computing, as other authors have already thoroughly covered this ground. Rather, it is an attempt to provide an introduction to the main areas of importance in a readable form. In addition, some basic details of the main clinical systems, as well as some of the smaller ones, are provided. The final chapter is on the use of PCs in general practice.

This book is aimed primarily at all those practice members who wish to know more about practice computing. Although some of the content is aimed at those considering a change of system, it is also intended for all those who simply want to do more with their existing system. I hope that it is of value to all of them.

Suffolk, 1999   A. J. R.

Acknowledgements

The list of people who have commented and suggested improvements to the text is long, and it would be impractical to mention all of them here. Of particular note, however, are the following:

Firstly, Dr Peter Orton who originally encouraged me to write this book. He has been a source of constant encouragement to me, making helpful suggestions and comments at every stage.

Secondly, and for the biggest contribution, I must thank my business partner and friend, Dr Tony Bowring, who has also been tireless in his reading and re-reading of the drafts. The final product is much improved by his useful suggestions and input.

Thirdly, to my publisher, Dr Peter Clarke and my editor, Richard Powell, at Petroc Press, and all those members of the industry who have commented on the chapters relevant to their systems.

Fourthly and finally, enormous thanks to Enn, my wife, who has had to put up with me during the time that I have been writing this book. She has made a major contribution by acting as a devil's advocate and reviewing the text from a non-technical point of view. Many passages have been revised in the light of her comments to make them more accessible to non-computer users.

1
Introduction to General Practice Computing

Opening Summary

This chapter introduces the topic of general practice computing with discussion of the benefits to GPs, staff and patients. It discusses the uses of general practice systems and the common hardware configurations. The basic elements of a computer are also covered.

Introduction

The use of computers by GPs has been steadily increasing over the last few years so that, at the time of writing, over 80% of practices have a practice computer system. Perhaps only half of these use their system to anything like its full potential. In the last 10 years developments in computer hardware have been truly staggering. Performance of CPUs – the main processing unit (or 'chip') in a computer – has increased by approximately a thousandfold. The cost per megabyte (Mb) of hard disk space had fallen from about £25/Mb in 1987 to approximately 3p/Mb in 1998. In 1987 a 'large' hard disk unit might have had a capacity of 20 Mb, whereas in 1998 6000 Mb (6 Gb) was commonplace. Typically, a powerful computer in 1986 might have had 0.5 Mb of random access memory (RAM). In 1998 even the most basic machines were equipped with 32 Mb, with 64 Mb or 128 Mb much more common.

Along with the increase in the power of PCs has been an increase in the records that necessarily must be kept by GPs. Most practices are now involved in some form of health-promotion activity and keep records of both their cytology and childhood immunisation targets. Certain groups of patients may be targeted with protocols of care, i.e. asthmatics. Health authorities are increasingly using GP links for registration changes and items of service claims. The advent of PCGs will probably increase the pressure still further. Trying to keep up with even these most basic requirements without using a computer is becoming more and more difficult. Modern systems will, of course, do a great deal more, and that is what this book is all about....

So what are the benefits of using a general practice system? These can be summarised as follows:

- Ease of routine administrative operations.
- Ease of authorised practice staff in accessing information.
- Bulk reporting.

The Benefits of General Practice Computing

We will now look at these categories in more detail.

Ease of Routine Administrative Operations

Many operations that form part of general practice are well defined and are the same for large groups of patients. Operations that fall into this category include issuing repeat prescriptions, data for heath promotion and target data. It is without question easier to carry out and record these operations using a good computer system than to do the job manually.

Ease of Authorised Practice Staff in Accessing Information

If a comprehensive medical record is maintained on the computer system then it is both more portable and more secure than the equivalent Lloyd George or A4 record. In a 'manual practice' it is always necessary for the staff to pull notes for patients attending surgeries. If a patient rings, for, say, a blood test result, many GPs will often want to have a look at the notes before responding. In a practice that keeps comprehensive notes on the computer, GPs can look at the patients' records on any convenient terminal, even when they are not in their consulting rooms.

Additionally, the computerised record is much more secure than the manual one. With a good computer system, even if the main computer is stolen and removed from the surgery, a thief would find it difficult to access patient records without the appropriate passwords. Also, provided that a backup has been taken, a GP can reload this on to a replacement computer and carry on business as usual. In a fully manual practice, not only are stolen patient records highly insecure, but also the GPs are left with inadequate information on which to base their care.

Bulk Reporting

Notwithstanding the above two categories, it is in the area of bulk reporting that computers have traditionally been recognised as being superior to manually based record systems. It is difficult to extract information on, for example, the number of patients with asthma, from the manual record system without employing some additional paper-based index. If the information has been entered in a suitable form onto the computer, then it is readily available in a short time. Another obvious example of this would be when a drug is recalled. In a manually based prescribing system, identifying all the people on a particular drug can be time consuming and difficult to achieve with total accuracy. On a properly based computerised system it is normally very easy to produce this information. The increasing use of audit in general practice only serves to emphasise this point.

The Benefits of Practice Computerisation for Staff, GPs and Patients

The benefits of a properly configured and operated general practice system differ, depending on your perspective. It is useful to look at how the prime benefits of using general practice systems vary according to the particular group that is considering them.

Benefits to GPs

From the points of view of GPs, the 'convenience' benefit, provided sufficient information exists on the computer, is very significant. If they need to ring a patient the registration details will contain the contact phone number. In a well-designed system the main events in the patient's clinical history can be very quickly assimilated from any point in the practice where there is a screen, and, in some cases, from the GP's home.

Certain groups of patients are recognised as needing regular reviews in order to control their medical conditions. Diabetics, hypertensives and asthmatics are three examples of these groups. A properly organised computer system will not only ensure that *all* the correct data is gathered, but will also issue a reminder that a review of a particular patient is due.

The value of having an infinite set of disease registers is more important to some GPs than to others, but most would agree that it is useful to be able to extract from the computer a list of patients who are suffering from a specified condition. It should be said that, even with the best of general practice systems, actually achieving this requires considerable planning and forethought.

Prescribing via the computer is often quoted as being a benefit to GPs of using a system. This is true for repeat prescriptions, where it is almost certainly quicker, once the system is set up, to issue them in this way. In terms of time taken, it is questionable as to whether writing an acute prescription by hand or issuing it from the computer is quicker. Clearly, other benefits derive from using the computer, such as maintaining a complete database of drugs issued and, on some systems, warnings of contraindications and possible harmful interactions with drugs already issued.

Various types of links are now possible between general practice systems and other computers. Both registration links and Items of Service (IOS) links have some benefit for GPs, but the real benefits are in practice administration. The most obvious links that directly benefit a GP are electronic pathology, where test results are sent directly from the laboratory to the general practice system and, in most cases, they are matched to the appropriate patient record. The new proposed Email links will also be beneficial. These will allow the GP to receive, for example, discharge notes directly from the hospital both quickly and in a clearly legible form.

Finally, another way in which general practice systems can be of benefit is in their reporting. GPs nowadays are ever more involved in carrying out audit, and clearly this is an activity where the computer can be of central benefit provided, as ever, that the data has been entered correctly on to the system in the first place.

Benefits to the Practice Team as a Whole for Administration

Many areas of practice administration involve carrying out clearly defined and repetitive tasks, and it is for this reason that computer systems have been most successful.

It is demonstrably easier for nurses and practice staff to record both smears and smear results on the computer, but to let the system check that the practice is on target for the next period (or to check the computations of the HA).

To a large extent, IOS claims can, when actioned via the computer, be automated and save an enormous amount of time over maintaining lists and filling out forms. If IOS links are in place, the savings can be even greater.

Most computer systems make it easy to identify groups of patients by running searches. Output from a search can usually be split into bands by age, etc. Similarly, changing all the patients on medication x to medication y can be a nightmare for practices if this has to be carried out manually, whereas it can be a five-minute operation on some general practice systems.

Many practices need to be able to analyse their referrals by such parameters as hospital and consultant. This may become more important when PCGs are fully established. This job is possible manually using a ledger, perhaps with a page for each consultant, and by adding referrals to the relative page. Implied in this is not just the actual time spent writing in the ledger but also in the collecting of the information. If the amount of time spent analysing the results is then considered, it is clearly better to enter referrals on the computer, *preferably* at the time of referral when analysis is often a matter of selecting an item from a menu and letting the computer do all the work.

Appointment systems are one area where most practices would see significant gains in efficiency provided the program used were to be both fast and easy to use. Paradoxically, in spite of this, most practices seem to find it useful to retain a manual system in some form.

Although audit is primarily a responsibility of GPs and nurses, practice staff are often involved in the extraction of data, and so the fact that computer systems allow bulk data to be analysed quickly, in most cases relieves the pressure. Such items as the practice annual report are made somewhat easier to compile if most of the required data is easily accessible.

The use of General Practice–Health Authority (GP–HA) links for the transfer of registration data (and in some cases IOS claims) has become widespread. Links of this kind are beneficial to both the practice and the HA, saving both practice time and leading to the more efficient management of registration data. However, some practices are still concerned about the security aspects of these links.

Benefits to Patients

Most of the benefits that accrue to patients of their GPs being computerised have already been mentioned, but it is worthwhile to consider which of these specifically affect patients.

Using a computer imposes constraints on a GP, but this can be a benefit to patients in as much as the record is more legible and often more structured, making it easier for the different health professionals to spot all of the relevant information quickly.

Prescribing is also easier, with much less room for error and a quicker service for patients, irrespective of whether 'their' GP is present or not. Patients are often less able to gain access to unnecessary repeats as many systems will indicate prescribing usage when a repeat is issued. A very high consumption is therefore, in principle, much easier to note.

The improvement in the monitoring of, for example, diabetic patients, which comes as a product of using templates, has benefits for patients as well as their GPs. They can expect to be monitored in a more consistent fashion than would otherwise be the case, with problems being recognised at an earlier stage. Using protocols on the computer developed by the GPs, nurses can take over more patient encounters while being confident that they are following practice policy in the treatment of the particular condition.

Cervical smear and other recalls, when carried out via the computer, are less likely to allow people to be forgotten owing to the degree of automation in the recall system and the reduction in the scope for human error. This particularly applies to patients who have not responded to standard health authority recalls. Of course, as always, this depends on the fact that the computer system is both easy to use and flexible to the needs of the practice.

Increasingly, one of the areas which is likely to lead to the biggest benefit for patients is that which involves links between the general practice system and other computer systems. In the future it is quite possible that appointments to secondary care will be able to be made while the patient is having the consultation with the GP, thus avoiding lengthy delays. The increase in access which secondary care will have to patients' primary care records, and vice versa, should lead to a situation where a more co-ordinated approach to health care can be made.

Telemedicine

Finally, the advent of remote conferencing into medicine brings the possibility of patients being examined by specialists at their own surgery when the specialist is physically elsewhere. Developments in conferencing software and hardware allow small video cameras and microphones to be linked to the computer. In this way consultations can be held remotely with examination of the patients being possible using remote 'gloves' linked using technology developed for virtual reality.

Simple video cameras are now available for PCs for about £100.

The History of Primary Care Computing

During the late 1980s the IBM PC became widely available, and suddenly there was a computer which really was a practical proposition as the basis of a working general practice system. Early systems were very basic compared to today's hardware. Hard disk units were uncommon and so most software needed to run from a floppy disk drive. However, experience was gained, and early versions of the most common software running today started to appear in the mid- to late-1980s.

One of the earliest initiatives was a scheme called 'Micros for GPs'. This was a Department of Health scheme to equip all practices with a microcomputer. Although its success was limited, many GPs were started on the road to practice computing in this way. Other schemes were run by some of the drugs companies.

Early systems were based around electronic prescribing, as this was the most easily identifiable area within the GPs' work that could be computerised. The idea of the paperless practice was a long way off.

Modern general practice systems have become possible owing to the rise of the small business computer. The first small easy-to-use machine was probably the Apple II, which apppeared around 1983, and a number of early primitive general practice record systems were written to run on this hardware.

The first systems to go into widespread use were produced by VAMP and AAH Meditel. Most people undertook to use the systems on the basis that they would be able to sell 'anonomised' patient data back to the supplier and so offset the cost of the system. In reality these schemes were not terribly successful, but they did have the effect of establishing both of these companies as major suppliers of general practice systems, a position they both still hold today.

Background to Current Systems

Over a hundred different general practice systems have been offered for sale at some time or another, but only about 25 of these are currently offering a product for sale. Since the advent of the Requirements for Accreditation (RFA) rules this number of suppliers has been steadily declining. The RFA rules are a basic specification for the functionality of a general practice system. In order for systems to be approved, suppliers submit their systems for testing to the appropriate body and the system is evaluated. The requirements (which form a lengthy document) are gradually being extended (in much the same way as the MOT test for cars is now rather more thorough than it was originally) to include new areas such as general practice links.

Suppliers *must* have their systems accredited in order that GPs can receive reimbursement from their HA. If a GP acquires a system which is not accredited, then reimbursement by the HA will not normally be made. While some flexibility has been shown in the past, the rules on this are now being tightened up and will be enforced much more rigorously in the future.

Suppliers generally divide into those that are 'large' and those that are not. The larger suppliers are generally considered to be more stable. So far smaller suppliers have generally managed to produce most of the more innovative software – as well as the worst. Table 1.1 sums up some of the points for and against each, although it should be stressed that these points are only generalisations.

The majority of the current suppliers use a turnkey approach and will supply a complete system. This comprises hardware, software and full installation, including integration of the age–sex register download from the HA. This makes the technical side of installing a system easier for the practice, but generally means that higher prices are paid for the hardware elements of the system. The advantage of acquiring this type of system is that if anything goes wrong all the support and maintenance should only be a 'phone call away – in theory, at least!

Table 1.1   Points for and against large and small suppliers

Large supplier	Smaller supplier
More stable	Less financial stability
Offer good support with helplines; open long hours	Help should be of a high quality – often from the software developer, but may be difficult to contact
The larger the installed user base, the greater the inertia to making small changes to the system	Developer can quickly incorporate a good idea from a user
Large suppliers have good hardware-support arrangements	Hardware support from the supplier can be limited, and slower
Large suppliers may have very busy helplines during normal hours making it difficult to get through	A small number of users means fewer people trying to obtain help
Maintenance income of the large installed base means that the future is more secure	Smaller income from maintenance makes it desirable for developers to be involved in other markets as well

General practice software is unlike ordinary business software in a number of ways. It normally has a tiny number of users when compared with even the smaller business programs. This means that, as well as having a much higher unit cost, the developer must find other sources of income. The main additional source of income within the general practice market is maintenance.

Users of general practice software, it is fair to say, often need rather more support than users of, for example, a word processing program. The costs of support and maintenance can be very large such that, over a period of years, the capital costs are less significant than the maintenance costs. This topic will be developed in the next chapter.

Another major difference between normal commercial software and general practice software is that, for example, one word processing package can often accept data from another. Further, in the case of spreadsheets, Microsoft Excel can understand a spreadsheet created in the rival Lotus 123 package.

In the case of general practice software, this is currently not the case. Data in one system cannot easily be transferred to another when patients move between GPs. Currently often the best that can be done is to export data as an 'ASCII' file (a standard format text file) that is in a form that can be used on a normal business PC. The increased use of Read-coded data is helping to alleviate this problem.

Basic Uses of General Practice Computer Systems

Although any delineation of functions on a general practice system is somewhat arbitrary, it is possible to divide up common functions into those which should probably be used initially by all practices and those which would normally only come into use later. This topic will be further developed in a later chapter.

The basic uses are:

- Registration
- Repeat prescriptions
- Cytology
- Childhood immunisations
- Health promotion projects
- Simple searches
- Registration links (for a suitably equipped practice)

Clearly the most basic use of any system is for the storing and manipulation of registration data, and this is logically the first part of the system that will be brought into use. This is made easier by the fact that, as previously mentioned, in most cases the patient data held by the HA will be imported into the system. Thorough checking of this imported data is necessary.

Existing repeats can take some time to set up from scratch, but in most cases the saving in time and effort from this point on makes the whole operation worthwhile. The above implies that the practice enters all the repeats on to the system quickly, but the actual method may well vary from practice to practice. Some will find it easier only to have a repeat put on when a new one is authorised, and although it may then take considerably longer to arrive at a complete dataset, the stress may be much less. Another method is to do all of the A's first and then all of the B's later, but the disadvantage of this method is that if the whole process takes some time, it can run out of steam and never become a complete record.

Without question it makes the job of whoever is responsible for cytology target information easier if the information is input into the computer as soon as possible. The benefits of having access to standard target reports make this job relatively attractive. In almost all cases the person who carried it out should also enter the smear on the computer. Administrative staff often enter results, although an easier and more efficient way is to receive the results from the laboratory electronically, if this service is available. The same comments also apply to childhood immunisation data as apply to smears.

The requirement for GPs to collect basic health data acted as a great stimulus for them to computerise. It is very difficult to collect data for projects without using a computer, but collecting the data can cause many problems if it is not gathered *with careful reference to the coded items which will be reportable*. We will also look into this area in some detail in a later section.

Virtually as soon as a practice starts to use a computer system the system becomes useful for simple searches. Perhaps the simplest (and initially the most reliable) ones that can initially be carried out are those on registration data, which can be very useful to a practice. In addition to these, the practice will soon need to learn how to run the standard searches to extract the reports for the topics mentioned above. The the first more complex searches that a practice might undertake are those involving basic health data, often so as to check that a figure given by a standard report is accurate. Searches of this type are often composed of more than one criterion and might, for example, be to find the asthmatic patients aged between 35 and 44.

Advanced Uses of the System

In one sense, advanced use of general practice systems is anything not mentioned above, but topics would include the following:

- Mailings to patients
- Clinical consultation data
- Complex searches
- Audit
- Protocols and templates for care guidelines
- Use of data exported to PCs, etc
- Scanning hospital letters

Mailings would include all types of standard letters to patients – from a letter informing them that a smear was negative, to one inviting a group of patients with diabetes to a clinic. Letters to consultants with summary medical histories would also be included.

Clinical encounter data would encompass the whole area of the electronic medical record, but would focus on the recording of patient encounters with Read codes and free text.

Complex searches would include all those that have to be set up explicitly by the user and which involve many parameters and/or a complex output format.

The use of a computer for medical audit implies a system that is widely used to store data and one where the operators are well used to the search routines. Computers are very useful when undertaking some types of audit as a quick and (normally) accurate method of extracting data.

Templates are generally user-defined forms that are used to collect a certain dataset for patients suffering from a particular condition. They permit the rapid collection of data and ensure that the data so collected is consistent between individuals. Setting up templates, although dependent on the system in use, is sometimes a fairly complex task. The loose description of a protocol in the computer sense is a template that allows different questions/data to be asked/collected depending on the results of earlier questions. For example, a nurse running through an asthma protocol with a patient might be asked to enter the peak flow. Depending on the value entered, the program might then instruct her to give the patient some advice or else to refer them immediately to the GP.

The presentation options for reports from most clinical computer systems are still rudimentary compared to modern business programs. With most systems some facilities exist to export the data from the general practice system and import it to an application running on a PC. For example, some audits might be performed using the practice system and the results obtained as a series of numbers. If this report were then exported to a PC, it could be presented as a chart giving the same information, but in a much clearer and easy-to-digest form.

Types of Hardware

Before considering general practice systems in detail, it is important to be aware of some of the hardware considerations which apply to different systems.

Current general practice systems fall into two main types: *multi-user* systems and *networked* systems.

A multi-user system consists of *one* central computer connected to a multiplexer. The multiplexer can be thought of as a large junction box with plugs in it for printers and terminals. All the work occurs on the central computer and the terminals and printers connected to it simply act as input and output devices. The arrangement is sometimes considered to be a star arrangement with the main computer at the middle and the terminals at the periphery. AAH Meditel and VAMP (VAMP Medical) currently have systems that use this arrangement, which is shown in diagrammatic form in Figure 1. A variation on the normal multi-user set-up is to replace some of the terminals with PCs. This adds flexibility to the system, in that the PCs can be used either as stand-alone systems running business software or as 'dumb' terminals on the multi-user system. This arrangement is shown in Figure 2.

The other main type of system is the local area network (LAN). In this arrangement there is still a main computer but each screen on the system is actually a PC with its own processing power. The effect of this *for the user* is that data can be transmitted around the system much faster than is possible using a multi-user system. Further, as PCs can support graphics, the screen displays can be rather more sophisticated than is the case with a text-based terminal. A typical arrangement of a LAN-based system is shown in Figure 3.

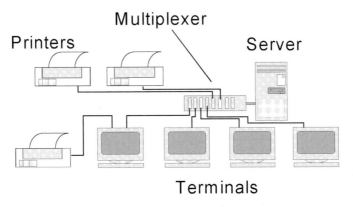

Figure 1   A typical multi-user system

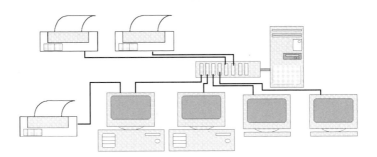

Figure 2   A multi-user system with PCs

Most of the computers in use in the UK today are IBM compatible. What IBM compatibility means in practical terms is that the computer has been designed with a certain set of rules in mind that will ensure that it is able to work with the vast majority of available software.

For the user the net effect of this is that, although it is very probable that the main computer of a general practice system will be IBM compatible, this is not so important, provided that it runs the clinical system software. What is important is that any computers (as distinct from 'dumb' terminals) attached to the system peripherally should be IBM compatible, as this will allow them to run the vast majority of non-clinical software.

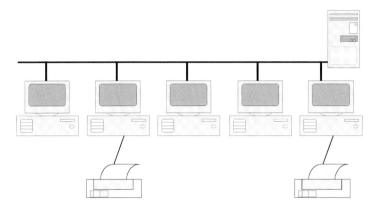

Figure 3   A typical network

More modern networks have wiring systems that resemble the multi-user system in Figure 2 but retain all the advantages of LANs.

Some suggestions for the technical specifications of system hardware are contained in the appendices, but a brief discussion of current specifications and terminology is relevant.

A Brief Guide to the Most Important Features of PCs

Many lengthy books have been written on the specifications of items of computer hardware. This section is designed to make the reader aware of some of the more important aspects to consider, and is by no means exhaustive.

Modern microcomputers are a collection of sub-systems. The main elements are as follows.

The Case

There are four basic sizes of case – desktop, mini tower, midi tower and tower. These come in two types – AT and ATX. The latter is relatively new and is starting to supersede the former, as it is has the advantage of having the expansion slots situated away from the central processing unit (CPU) so that expansion cards do not foul it.

The mini tower is probably currently the most popular configuration. It normally has dimensions of about 300 mm (height), 280 mm (depth) and 170 mm (width). It is designed either to stand upright beside the monitor or else on the floor or a shelf. The advantage of this type is that it is both reasonably small and has enough room inside for some expansion.

The desktop case has similar dimensions to the mini tower case but is designed to lie on its largest surface, underneath the monitor. Its chief advantage is that as the monitor screen is on top of it, the height is raised as well. Tower cases are normally used for fileservers and for other computers where a number of extra peripheral components, such as hard disks, CD-ROMs, tape back up units, etc need to be fitted into the case's bays. They are often 600–700 mm tall, and are more expensive than the other types.

The Keyboard

Keyboards are available from many suppliers, but most tend to be similar both in appearance and function. The exception to this is the 'new' Microsoft natural keyboard that has its keys arranged in a staggered 'V' configuration. This is meant to reduce the risk of users developing repetitive strain injury (RSI).

The main difference between keyboards is the feel of the keys. Some are designed to have a 'click' feel when keys are pressed, whereas others have none. Choosing a keyboard is a surprisingly personal decision, and having the 'right' keyboard can be very important for the user. The only safe way to obtain a satisfactory one is to try out the various types available. Replacement keyboards are an inexpensive option.

The Motherboard

At its most basic, the motherboard is the most important component in the computer and contains the central processing unit (CPU), the random-access memory (RAM) and, in some systems, the cache RAM, as well as all the support chipsets that comprise a functional unit. It also contains the expansion slots into which such items as sound cards and internal modems are inserted. One major difference between motherboards is the type of 'bus' in use. The bus is the electronic highway that connects different systems together, and historically it could be any of the following types: ISA, EISA, VL or PCI. Currently a PCI/ISA bus is the most desirable, for reasons beyond the scope of this book, but other bus technologies are now being released, such as the AGP and the USB.

The Processor – the CPU

The processor is the heart of the computer and has a major effect on how fast it operates. Ten years ago the CPUs used in PCs were 8-bit 8088/8086 types and computers containing these processors are still in use in business today – just. These were followed by the much more powerful 16-bit 80286 types (backwardly compatible with the previous 808X systems). The number of bits in the description of a processor can be loosely considered to be the number of 'lanes' for the manipulation of data and instructions – analogous to the lanes on a motorway. 80286 processors, although still in use, are utterly obsolete.

The next generation of processors were the 80386 types. The first was the 80386DX, which was closely followed by the less-sophisticated 80386SX. These also maintained backwards compatibility with the previous types and both were 32-bit externally, although the 80386SX type was only 16-bit internally.

These were succeeded by the again backwardly compatible 80486SX and 80486DX types. The terms SX and DX here have different meanings from their equivalents that were used for 80386 processors. An 80486DX has an on-board math's co-processor, which significantly speeds up intensive mathematical operations. This is absent or disabled in the 80486SX. Both of these processors are now obsolete, but are still being used for non-intensive applications. Many practices still have file servers, etc based on this type of processor.

The current processor of choice is the Pentium II, which is a much improved development of the 80486, and it is this type of processor that should be present inside any new computer. Intel produce the majority of these processors, but a number of other suppliers, such as Cyrix and AMD, produce equivalents at the lower end of the market. Currently most new computers contain Pentium II processors, although for basic tasks Pentium MMX (or equivalent) processors can be used.

As well as the *type* of processor used in a computer, the *speed* of the processor is also important. Speed is measured in MHz (megahertz – millions of cycles per second) and generally the higher the speed the better. Currently Pentium II chips are available in speeds of 233–450 MHz.

If the reader finds the above explanations to be too complicated, then accept that a Pentium 233 MHz processor is the lowest specification that should be considered in *any* new machine, with the 300 MHz Pentium II and above being suitable as fileservers.

RAM

RAM (random access memory) refers to the electronic memory fitted into a motherboard and is loosely equivalent to the electronic 'workspace' of the system. Another analogy would be to compare it with human memory. RAM is measured in megabytes (millions of bytes – Mb). A megabyte, very loosely speaking, is the amount of storage needed to store 500 pages of plain text.

The absolute minimum amount of memory acceptable in a sytem is 32 Mb, although a lot of modern applications require 64 Mb. If a number of Windows applications are to be used, 128 Mb is better and 256 Mb (or even more!) would be the optimum amount needed in a fileserver serving a network of 10–15 screens.

Cache

Most motherboards are designed to accept a small amount of special high-speed memory known as *cache*. This can have the effect of speeding up the machine for only a very modest extra investment. Cache memory is normally supplied in quantities of 256 kb (kilobytes – thousands of bytes), 512 kb or 1024 kb. The best current compromise between additional cost and performance in most machines is 512 kb. Pentium IIs have the cache built in.

Input/Output (I/O) Ports

The I/O ports are what the computer uses to communicate with other peripheral devices such as printers and mice. There are two basic types of ports – serial and parallel – the names describing how they transfer data. Parallel ports are normally used to connect to printers and sometimes to external tape back-up devices and scanners, while serial ports are normally used to connect to external devices such as mice, modems, etc. It is usual to have one parallel port and two serial ports on a computer, integrated on to the motherboard. Having only one serial port on the system can sometimes lead to problems, e.g. when a mouse and an external modem both need to be connected and there is no separate mouse port.

If you intend to use an external modem with a computer, it should have a *high speed* serial port for this purpose. All currently available models use this type as standard. New computers should ideally also be equipped with a universal serial bus (USB) port. This new type of port allows faster communication with peripheral hardware, although only a few compatible devices are currently available.

Hard Disk

The hard disk is the computer's permanent storage system. It stores both data and programs. If RAM is analogous to memory, then the hard disk is analogous to paper. It is the basic medium used to record information. The capacity of hard disk units, like RAM, is measured in megabytes (Mb). A small hard disk would currently store around 3 Gb (three gigabytes, equal to 3000 Mb), with 6 Gb being 'average'. New fileservers, no matter how small the practice, should be at least 6 Gb.

There are two different types of hard disk subsystems currently being manufactured, namely EIDE and SCSI. The latter give marginally faster access to the hard disk, faster data transfer and larger capacities. However, SCSI devices are somewhat more expensive than the equivalent EIDE ones.

Floppy Disks

A floppy disk drive unit is required so that data can be transferred to and from the computer. Both 5¼-inch and 3½-inch types are in use, but a new computer normally only needs to be supplied with a single 3½-inch drive. A new type of 3½-inch drive called the LS120 allows normal, as well as high capacity (120 Mb), floppy disks to be used.

Video Card

The video card (also called the *graphics* card) handles the electronic output from the CPU and converts it to a form that can be displayed on a monitor. Only a few years ago video cards were relatively unsophisticated, but now their development and manufacture has become an industry in its own right, with faster and faster cards producing higher and higher resolutions in millions of colours.

Video cards normally have their own fast memory and at least 2 Mb should be present if a high-resolution SVGA screen is to be used. Systems needing a large number of colours at high resolution may need cards fitted with 4 Mb or even 8 Mb of memory.

Monitor

Monitors are all made to operate to at least the minimum standard (VGA), but most conform to a higher specification (SVGA) and some to a higher specification still (XGA). They come in screen sizes of 12 inches to 27 inches, but the most popular sizes are now 15 inches and 17 inches. Monitors, like keyboards, are largely a matter of personal taste. Some of the very cheap unbranded monitors that are occasionally supplied by general practice system suppliers are of very low quality. If at all possible, specify a well-known brand such as NEC or Sony, and make sure that any monitors supplied conform to the MPRII standard for radiation emissions (virtually all monitors on the market do conform).

Operating Systems

All computers require an operating system before they can run any software at all. The operating system can be likened to the 'personality' of the computer and without it the hardware is useless. A good analogy is to compare people brought up in different parts of the world. They are all very similar physiologically, but they all speak different languages.

The most common operating system in the world is Windows 95 although MS-DOS and Windows 3.1 are still in widespread use. It is not particularly important which operating system your general practice system uses, but the attached PCs should be capable of running Windows 95/98, and computers not attached directly to the general practice system will normally be run under Windows 95/98.

Current operating systems in use include Windows 95/98, UNIX, MUMPS, DOS, XENIX, Pick and BOS. For new installations the last four of these operating systems are not recommended.

A detailed discussion of operating systems is not necessary here, but having a general practice system which is designed to run under Windows 95/98 is clearly an advantage when compared with a system running, say, XENIX. This is because the network and workstations can also be used to run ordinary commercial software.

Printers

It is appropriate at this point to discuss briefly the different types of printer that are available and their uses.

Dot matrix printers are both cheap and long lasting, and are quite suitable for general work such as FP10s and internal reports. The running costs are quite low, as the only consumables required are ribbons and paper. The only downside (apart from the noise) is that the quality of the print is not very high, although on modern machines it is quite readable.

Inkjet printers are more expensive than dot matrix ones, but produce a significantly better quality of print. They are more expensive to run and are generally a little more fragile mechanically (there is more to go wrong), but they can be used for high-quality correspondence, if necessary. Also, they offer the facility of printing in colour. Unfortunately only a very small number of inkjet printers can accept continuous paper for prescriptions, and most of these have now been discontinued.

Laser printers are potentially more expensive to buy, but produce excellent results and are not very much more expensive to run on a per page basis than dot matrix printers. They are also much quieter. Owing to the relatively high (but falling) initial cost, they are usually sited in the office and are used solely for correspondence and other work that needs to be of high quality. In the last few years many 'personal' laser printers have appeared on the market. Although these are not engineered for an office environment, they can offer excellent value for home or light use.

Colour printers are also available and some dot matrix and inkjet printers come with this option. Colour laser printers are not yet a practical proposition (on cost grounds), although they will be within the next few years. Most colour printers use sublimation techniques that make them costly and too specialised to be of interest in general practice, although the price of colour laser printers has fallen five-fold in the last three years.

Other Hardware

Modems are increasingly becoming standard pieces of equipment within general practice. They allow information from a computer to be transmitted via the telephone line so that it can be received by another modem attached somewhere else to the telephone network. They are often used where branch surgeries need to be linked to main surgeries and can also be used to connect the surgery to the HA, laboratory, or anywhere else. There is also a special type of modem that is used with high-speed digital telephone lines (a terminal adapter) that essentially does the same job – but much faster.

In the last few years there has been an explosion in the use of CD-ROMs in the computer industry. A computer CD-ROM is very like its audio equivalent, and allows large amounts of data to be stored on a single disk. The disks are normally read only – data cannot be written to them, but rewritable disks/disk writers are becoming increasingly available at constantly reducing prices.

A significant minority of practices are now paperless (approximately 10–15%) in that all clinical patient information is stored in the computer. However, the practices still receive large amounts of paper information about their patients. Summarised information can then be entered manually into the patient record and the paper letters either kept or scanned into the computer. The scanning option is still unusual, but people are increasingly looking for methods whereby paper documents can be scanned into the computer and therefore held in electronic form as part of the clinical record. This need not, contrary to popular opinion, be a very expensive option.

Closing Summary

This aim of this introductory chapter was to introduce the topic of general practice computing in an easily readable form. It has concentrated largely on the benefits of computerising and the processes involved, and finished by discussing the hardware associated with general practice systems.

The main benefits seen were discussed from the perspectives of

- *GPs*
- *Administration*
- *Patients*

It is hoped that the reader has been convinced of the benefits of the computerised approach, and we will now go on to consider in more detail the selection of a general practice system.

2
How to Select a General Practice System

Opening Summary

This chapter covers the logical approach to the selection of a general practice system. In particular, it will assist practices to be clear about their objectives and then to look at demonstrations of appropriate systems. Coding systems, and Read codes in particlar, are discussed in detail.

Assessing Aims

Before moving on to the actual selection of a general practice system, it is very important to have clearly defined objectives. These will depend on whether or not the practice already has a computer. Questions that should be asked include the following:

1. **In the first instance, is the system to be used ...**

(a) Primarily by staff?
If the answer is 'yes', is a fully featured clinical system necessary? Do the partners envisage using the system in consultations in the future? Clearly, if the system is to be used mainly as a back office system, it must allow the efficient input of the relevant data and the output of the necessary reports. Important areas include repeat prescribing management and the easy maintenance of immunisation and smear data.

(b) By staff and nurses?
If nurses are going to use the system, new patient checks should be easy to enter. In addition, a simple method of including the data on asthma, diabetes and CHD should be carefully considered, together with the nature and ease of production of reports on these groups and on basic health data.

(c) By all team members, including the GPs?
If all team members, including the GPs, are going to use the system, the clinical aspects of the medical records become overwhelmingly import-

ant, together with the easy issuing of acute and repeat prescriptions. The ability to search clinical data in a flexible way is also very significant.

2. What would be the principal benefits of a change of the existing computer?

(a) Easier operation...
If an existing system is being upgraded, it may well be possible to improve the user interface.

(b) More functionality...
Features such as easy searching, automatic checks on data entered, flexible methods of patient identification and better links to other computer programs such as word processing and spreadsheets.

(c) More speed...
Computer hardware developments have moved on at a much greater pace than software developments over the last few years. Consequently, if an old fileserver is replaced by a new one, it can cause a dramatic increase in speed of operation.

(d) Better expansion options in the future...
Quite a number of practices have had systems supplied by very small suppliers for a number of years. Often these systems were originally designed as electronic age–sex registers with prescribing. In some cases the supplier is not able to provide the general practice links options which are now becoming essential.

(e) Better support...
The quality of support varies widely from supplier to supplier. When upgrading it is essential to ascertain the quality, price and extent of the support that you can expect to receive.

(f) Lower costs...
Depending on the type of the present system and its proposed replacement, it is quite possible that a practice can upgrade to a superior and more functional system, while at the same time considerably reducing annual support costs.

3. What can sometimes be the disadvantages of a change in an existing system or the installation of a new one?

(a) Higher costs
For uncomputerised practices the capital costs of acquiring a new system can be very high. In addition to this, there will be maintenance

charges and perhaps training, if this is not all inclusive. For practices that are changing system, apart from the benefits, the downside is that the capital costs can be very significant, and in some areas HA reimbursement may not be forthcoming.

(b) More work – especially if full Lloyd George records are kept
When practices computerise, the amount of work inevitably rises, as manual systems have to be maintained. Even in practices which maintain comprehensive clinical records on the computer, it is currently normal for Lloyd George notes also to be kept up to date. Only on systems where a full audit trail is present can the maintenance of paper records be relaxed, and even in these cases there is still some doubt as to the legality of this approach (although an increasing number of practices are paperless).

(c) Training/retraining
Training key staff to use various parts of the computer system is relatively time-intensive. Usually, only a few selected members of the practice will attend the training sessions that are run by the supplier. Time then has to be found to train the remaining members of staff.

In a situation where staff are learning a new system, having already trained on a previous computer system, there may be considerable reluctance and resistance to retraining.

(d) Adaptation of practice systems to suit the computer system
Depending on the nature of the selected system, it may well be necessary to initiate changes in practice procedures to suit the system. For example, instigating a computerised repeat prescribing system will certainly affect the manual methods which patients and staff currently use. Converting manual disease registers is another example. These may be held on a card index system or may simply be a clinic list used by the nurse/GPs.

The successful implementation of a computer system in a general practice depends to a significant extent on how well the practice is managed manually. If a non-computerised practice has good manual systems that are enabling the practice to carry out its functions, it is likely that transferring some or all of these systems to a computer will be successful. If, on the other hand, the practice views the acquisition of a computer system as a method which will 'magically' solve all of its deficiencies and problems in terms of practice organisation and management, it is unlikely that the implementation of a computer system will *significantly* improve the situation. In this situation the only benefit of computerisation is likely to be in areas such as repeat prescribing, where the very structures imposed by using the computer to carry out this task may lead to an improvement.

When setting objectives it is unlikely that it will be possible to find a system which satisfies all the objectives completely. For this reason prioritisation is important. For example, a practice may well wish to reduce ongoing costs and to find a system that allows the issue of repeat scripts with as few keystrokes as possible. It may well turn out that the objectives are to some extent mutually exclusive – particularly the cost versus features situation.

In the implementation of large-scale database systems in commerce, significant time is devoted to 'systems analysis'. This is the process by which the proposed database is matched to the needs and goals of the proposed users. Although it is unlikely that any practice nowadays will have a system specifically developed for them, many of the same techniques can still be used.

All of the relevant staff should be involved in the process, as simply imposing a system on them is rarely successful. From each individual's requirements, some idea of the ideal system can be ascertained. It should not be thought that those who lack expertise in computer systems are unable to contribute to this process. As an example, a nurse who keeps a card index manual record of the asthmatics in a practice has a clear idea of the data that should be stored, as well as the information required for reports. If a system fails to allow an important item of information to be stored easily, it can have a very negative effect on what was previously a successful manual data-handling operation.

It appears that in many practices systems have been acquired in a casual and haphazard manner – often under pressure exerted by external bodies. It is absolutely vital that the whole process of selection and implementation of the practice computer system is given as much consideration as possible.

Consider now the following scenarios....

New System...

'We never seriously considered buying a computer until last year because the practice seemed to be producing all the information required. We were achieving the higher targets for immunisations and cytology. So why spend the money...?

Then the health authority said that provided we chose a system by 31/03/XX we could have it at ninety percent reimbursement – oh, and we would get a link to them which would allow us to keep our patient registrations up to date. The partners discussed this at their weekly meeting in early March and I was requested to seek the advice of the health authority on acquiring a system. In the end we attended a road show in a hotel where about four systems were set up. As we only had five days left to get the 90% deal, we went for the same system that most of the other practices there were buying.

We did have a demonstration but it only lasted for about 20 minutes and it is difficult to take things in. Unfortunately, as far as I can remember, none of the areas in which we have problems were actually shown to us.

Since the system was installed we have had nothing but problems. All the extra work has meant we have now slipped below the higher target level for smears. We found out that when the system was being used in surgery it took at least four minutes to set up a repeat and then while it was printing the whole screen would freeze.

The partners are so angry that the system does not work in consultations (that part has not been developed yet), that they have stopped using it! I've seen some other systems now but I do wish we had been able to take a little more time in selecting our system.

I'm sorry I can't talk for any longer but due to the fact that the staff had the new system imposed on them both our senior receptionists have left and I'm about to do an interview....'

Upgrade from the Existing System...

'We had an XXXX system for some years and in many ways it led to an improvement in several of the practice information systems. We used it mainly for repeat prescribing and targets, although we had started to put some other clinical information on to it. Last year we decided to have a look at other systems. The practice manager arranged demos of all the leading systems, to take place on Wednesday afternoons. Unfortunately, on most occasions a number of the partners could not attend the demonstration. On average, just the practice manager and a different GP were present at each demonstration. All the systems looked very good, but it was difficult to appreciate the strengths and weaknesses of each one. After five demonstrations we were all confused as to which system was which. Anyway, time went on and then we received a mailing from one of the companies offering a 25% reduction in price if we signed up within seven days. So we did.

The company promised to convert all the data from our old system but it did not use Read codes. All the data has been converted to free text in the new system. This cannot be searched and it meant that all the target and health promotion data had to be re-entered. The prescribing was converted to the new system but for some technical reason all the acutes on the old system became repeats overnight. We are sorting out the problems but it has caused everyone a lot of work.

Overall the new system is much better than the old one but there are a number of areas that are not as good. If we ever change system again we will be a lot more careful....'

The above examples illustrate what can happen if a computer system is implemented in a haphazard fashion, and each scenario is based on many occurrences of similar events.

We will now discuss the issues in more detail.

Coding Systems

Many GPs and practice staff are confused by the whole issue of coding systems in computer software. *The implementation of the coding system* **(which should be Read codes for all new systems**) *is one of the most important distinguishing features between different systems.*

Consider the simple term *diabetes mellitus*. If this morbidity is stored in the clinical record of a patient on a computer system it can be stored in one of two ways:

- As a coded item – the term can be selected from a *dictionary* of terms.
- As free text – the term can be recorded in a unstructured text field.

The problem with the latter approach is that inconsistency and human error can lead to the term being recorded in a variety of ways, e.g.:

Diabetes Mellitus
Diabetes mellitus
diabetes mellitus

or even...

Diabetis Mellatus
etc, etc, etc

Searching free text fields using a computer system is often an inefficient process, assuming that the facility exists at all. Normally the lack of consistency in the data entered renders the process useless for extracting, for example, a list of those patients who are suffering from a specified condition.

Various coding systems have been used to code morbidity, symptoms, actions, etc since clinical computer systems first became widespread. Some of the more popular methods are shown below. Coding systems are either *flat* or *hierarchical*. Flat systems give equivalent codes for all coded items, whereas hierarchical systems have an inverted tree-like structure with a main *high level* code representing the most general form of the condition and *subcodes* of this code representing specific instances.

Arbitrary

A flat coding system in which the user defines the term which can then be picked from a list. This is much better than using free text but is entirely local to the practice. Management of the system can become difficult if a large number of codes are required, and different codes for the same condition can be entered accidentally.

RCGP

A coding system originated by the body of the same name. A numerically based system with terms defined for each code. The system is essentially flat with some hierarchical elements. Used in the AMC (now part of AAH Meditel) and several other systems until Read codes were introduced.

ICD9, ICD10

A system widely used in hospitals with some hierarchical elements. Historically this system was used by a number of general practice systems, but has now been overtaken by Read codes.

OXMIS

A flat system which found favour with the first-generation general practice systems. Still widely used by VAMP Medical Practices as well as the Update system now owned by Torex.

Read

The preferred system for current general practice systems (for systems to be accredited, and hence attract reimbursement, they must use the Read coding system). This system is fully hierarchical and both four-digit and five-digit versions are in use.

Read Codes

Read codes were originally designed by James Read and have been adopted by the NHS as the standard coding system for use throughout the health service The codes consist of up to five characters which can all be alphanumeric.

Taking the example of diabetes mellitus:

> This has the Read code C10.., and is a *high level* code. It is made up as follows starting from the left:

C – the highest level code representing endocrine, nutritional, metabolic and immunity disorders
C1 – a *subcode* of the above representing endocrine gland diseases other than thyroid gland disorders
C10 – a subcode of the above representing diabetes mellitus

The term *diabetes mellitus* has a large number of sub-terms lower in the hierarchy describing more specific situations, i.e.:

C107 – Diabetes mellitus with peripheral circulatory disorder

This term also has sub-codes, such as:

C1072 – Diabetes mellitus adult with gangrene

which is a full five-digit code at the bottom of the hierarchy with no further detail possible (at the present)

Users can use as detailed a code as they wish, with the overwhelming advantage that most of the diabetic codes start with C10. A search for this should capture patients with any subcodes.

For those readers who have a four-digit Read-coded system, it should be pointed out that four-digit Read codes follow the same system but with only a maximum of four digits being available. Within the four-digit Read codes some items have different high-level codes, i.e. diabetes mellitus is not C10.. but C2.. A new version of the Read codes will soon be available and this will allow users to specify an item in even more detail.

Even though the above example used a morbidity to illustrate the coding system, it should not be assumed that Read coding is limited to such items. Illness and disease are just one section (or chapter) of the Read system, and others exist for such areas as occupations, history/symptoms, examination/signs, laboratory procedures, etc.

Faced with such a vast number of codes, new users to a Read-coded system can have a lot of difficulty finding the code they need – or even deciding between a number of options. Normally, users do not have to remember codes as they are entered using the *rubric*, i.e. to enter the C10.. code you might type in DIABET, when prompted. The screen will then show a list of codes with rubrics starting in DIABET. You can descend (or ascend) through the Read hierarchy until the desired code is found. If you *do* know the code, then it is often very much quicker to use it rather than go though lists of codes.

It should be stressed that the implementation of Read codes in a system is a very important factor to consider if GPs are intending to use the system in consultation. Accreditation has placed some requirements on to system suppliers, but there are still wide variations in the nature of the user interface.

Occasionally, in spite of the vast number of Read codes provided, a user will not be able to find a code to cover a particular situation. In this instance some systems will allow the user to add user-defined codes to the appropriate part of the Read system. An alternative approach is to apply to the National Coding Centre in order to have the required code added to the system. Strategies for using Read codes are discussed further in Chapter 4.

Choosing a Shortlist of Computer System Suppliers

There are a relatively large number of general practice system suppliers and it would be impracticable for most practices to look at all of the systems that are available.

In Chapter 1 we looked at the relative merits of choosing a system from a large supplier versus a small supplier, and some of the other fundamentals of choosing a system.

Probably for most practices it is sensible to look at a shortlist of about four or five systems which have been chosen because they appear to offer the system that the practice requires.

There are various ways of selecting systems for the shortlist, including the following.

Users' Input

As previously mentioned, all the users of a system should have a major input into the selection at each stage of the process. It should be possible for each member of the practice to list their most important requirements and then for these individual requirements to be turned into a practice list against which systems can be measured.

The NHS training division has produced a toolkit providing questionnaires that could be useful in this respect (see under Further Reading for more details).

Clearly, those practices that already have a computer system are in a better position than those that do not. As well as being able to list their requirements, they should also be able to express their views on how particular functions should, or should not, be implemented. As an example....

> ...In a particular general practice system that was in use a few years ago, the user, when issuing repeats, had to select all the items *not* required. This meant that for a patient who needed one item out of half a dozen, numerous keystrokes were required to deselect all the others. This feature drove the staff

> of some practices to distraction in busy periods, and when these practices changed their systems, careful attention was paid to the layout and operation of this task.

Published Reviews

Published reviews of systems can help in the selection. They can provide a comparison of features between systems as well as commenting on typical system costs and the package as a whole. They can be found in the mainstream general practice weeklies such as *Pulse* and *GP* and in *Practice Computing*, which appears quarterly.

In-practice Knowledge

It may well be that staff or partners of a practice have had experience of other systems in the past and this working experience can be put to good use. It is a definite advantage when selecting a system to have a practice member who is familiar with the system in question.

The opposite view, however, is that some GPs and staff have too much enthusiasm for systems that they have previously used and that this enthusiasm may not be entirely justified. The situation can be analogous to the 'my car is the best car in the world' syndrome. On balance, however, previous knowledge should give a definite plus to a system when the choice has been narrowed down to two or three possible contenders.

Local Practices

Local practices can be a useful source of information when looking for a system and they are discussed in a later part of this section. However, be aware that, although you can probably find out from other users if a system is truly unsatisfactory, the 'my car is the best car in the world' syndrome still applies if the practice perceives that the system is working well.

Dispensing Status

If a practice is dispensing, then the question of the computerisation of this function needs to be raised. It is probably true that the general practice system with the best overall dispensing features is not so good in other areas. Some good general practice systems do not offer dispensing features at all and others use a bought-in module which is not well integrated with the rest of the system. If, after careful thought, the practice wants a system which can handle stock control and automatic reordering, the choice of systems on offer becomes much smaller. Another approach might be to separate the two functions and acquire a dispensing control system via one of the big drug companies while having a non-dispensing general practice system. However, it should be pointed out that most of the general practice systems that could be described as non-dispensing still have a facility to print labels for prescriptions and this may satisfy the needs of some practices.

Financial Factors

Some years ago there was a considerable difference in cost between most of the 'small' system suppliers and the larger system suppliers. That difference has since diminished, so that nowadays it is easy to pay somewhat more for a system from one of the small suppliers than a larger one. Notwithstanding, if cost is a major factor, then some of the smaller suppliers will be able to supply a system for considerably less hard cash. It is important however to compare like with like and a system which appears cheaper at the first instance can end up costing more before it is fully functional. In particular, with some of the larger suppliers everything you might wish for is included in the quoted price (i.e. accounts software, template designer, etc) whereas these are chargeable separately in other cases.

Clinical or Administrative Systems

These will have a major bearing on cost as a system that is not installed in the consulting rooms needs rather less hardware. It will, however, have rather less function and the cost of extending the system into a full clinical system in the future should be born in mind.

Multiple Sites

If the practice has more than one site, a decision will have to be taken as to whether to computerise one or more of them. If more than one site is to be computerised, the normal solution would be to install a dedicated landline between the sites. This solution, although normally effective, is costly both in terms of installation and rental. Another possibility for a site that is not used intensively is to use an ordinary telephone line and a pair of modems, which is much cheaper than a dedicated landline. The final option is to computerise initially on one site only and to accept that a manual system must be maintained in some form to deal with the other site(s). Some form of encounter sheet can often be employed to gather data at the uncomputerised site.

If a landline or modems are to be employed, it is essential that the supplier concerned has adequate experience of the technologies involved. It is always worth requesting a visit to another practice using this supplier's system before proceeding.

Supplier Demonstrations

Demonstrations are an important aspect of selecting a general practice system, but in many cases practices fail to reap the full benefit from them. This section attempts to describe how to achieve the most out of supplier demonstrations.

Arranging Demonstrations

If at all possible, demonstrations should be arranged at the practice for all the systems in which the practice is interested. It is most important to arrange the time so that all the relevant personnel can be present. Often members of the practice have to cancel at short notice (for quite understandable reasons, such as an urgent home visit, etc). This is unfortunate for the practice as well as being frustrating for the system supplier, who may have travelled a long way to do the demonstration. For these reasons they should be arranged on a day when

- All of the intended attendees can be present.
- Most of the partners are available. If necessary, use locum cover.
- Sufficient time will be available for the demonstration and for questions afterwards.

Taking Charge of the Session

Many demonstrations proceed in a manner something like the following:

- The representative welcomes the opportunity to display his company's system and proceeds to go through a set-piece demonstration of the system in question.
- The practice personnel listen, but make few comments.
- The representative finishes the demonstration and offers to send in a quotation for a system.
- They then leave.

The following approach would be better....

- The representative proceeds to go through a set-piece demonstration of the system.
- The practice members listen, but interrupt when they require clarification of any point.
- Everyone makes brief notes on the system, highlighting both the good and the bad points, as they perceive them to be.
- At the end of the formal demonstration the practice manager asks if he/she can enter some data appropriate to one of his/her colleague's job. *It is very important that individuals actually use a system rather than simply having it demonstrated to them.* The number of keystrokes and the time taken is much more apparent than is the case when simply watching a demonstration. Representatives will often be uncomfortable with this approach, and may well be ill equipped to deal with it, but persist, as it will pay dividends.
- The representative finishes, offers to send in a quotation for a system and then leaves. The practice then spends 10 or 15 minutes discussing the system and scoring it against their requirements.

Using this technique in demonstrations is certainly more difficult (and a lot more like hard work!), but the selected system may be in use for many years, and to adapt an old adage 'select in haste repent at leisure'. The basic idea is to be in control of the session and to ask the representative to show you what you want to see. Sometimes they will not be able to answer all your questions. If they promise to 'get back to you' and then fail to so, you can deduce the support that you might well expect from this company. Bear in mind that demonstration systems often have very few patients on them, and so searches appear to be both fast and easy!

Other Methods of Viewing Systems

There are a number of ways of viewing systems, other than the demonstration mentioned above:

- Visits to exhibitions
- Visits to other practices
- Borrowing a system

Visits to Exhibitions

As the sole method of selecting a system, visits to exhibitions are inadequate. However, to obtain some feeling for particular systems, they are ideal. HAs often set up bulk demonstrations with five or six suppliers present. Individual suppliers periodically demonstrate to all comers at roadshows – often held in hotels. Finally, various groups often have supplier demonstrations attached to their events. One example of this would be the annual meeting of the British Computer Society, Primary Health Care Group.

Perhaps the greatest benefit of this type of event is the ability to compare different systems *at the same time*. It is quite feasible to spend 15 minutes looking at, for example, the clinical data entry screen of one system and then walk across a room and look at the same part of another system.

Perhaps the only danger of events of this type is the temptation to sign up to a particular system while still in the first flush of enthusiasm!

Visits to Other Practices

Visits to practices are also extremely useful in order to gain information on a particular system of interest. Practices already using a system can give you very valuable information on how a particular system actually works in reality. They can also give a realistic estimate of the quality of the support. Whereas in the case of system demonstrations it is important that the whole practice team sees the system at the same time (anything else would be impractical), it is often better in the case of a practice visit for different team members to visit the other practice individually. In this way they can gain an in-depth understanding of how this particular system will affect them in relation to their own jobs.

Borrowing a System

If the process of selection has led to one particular system being favoured, then it can be very useful to borrow a system from the supplier for a short time. This is so that those key members of the practice staff can go through the system to make sure that there are no hidden snags. Most suppliers will agree to this, provided they are confident that this will probably lead to a sale.

To borrow a system may seem like an unnecessary step to some readers, but I would stress that the greater the number of ways that you can use to assess a system *before* buying it, the better. In many of the practices that I visit in the course of my work, the staff wish that more time and effort could have been put into the selection of their particular practice computer system.

Other Considerations

As well as the functionality of the software, practices should consider a number of other factors in the selection of their practice software. In particular the overall costs of the system over a period of time should be compared to other systems. This cost is best calculated over a period of five years – the longest period of time that the system might be expected to function without significant upgrading. Items to consider include the cost of software and hardware, and any additional charges for accounts software or an appointment system. Some suppliers make a further charge for communications software for GP–HA links. Additionally there may be a data-conversion charge to cover the cost of converting data from a previous system, or an HA download charge to load the registration data into the system. Training may be separately chargeable, as, in a few cases, may be upgrades to the software. The costs of cabling should be considered. Additional miscellaneous smaller charges may be payable for a Read code site licence and for a wide area network (WAN) connection fee to connect a practice to the network that links them to the HA and to others. Finally, the costs of registering for data protection must be taken into account.

Support Record

To a large extent one must take the assurances of the supplier on trust with regard to the support that they give both over the phone and when necessary by visiting the practice. A simple way that can sometimes be used is to try out the support before the practice buys. This is particularly easy if the practice borrows a system. Simply ask for, and then call, the support line and assess how knowledgeable is the voice at the other end. Was the call answered promptly? Did they promise to ring back because all support lines were busy? Even if the practice has not borrowed a system you can still ask for the helpline number and ring it to clarify some aspect of the proposed system. If the salesman is reluctant to give the helpline number before you order a system, you should draw your own conclusions.

It is also worth looking at reviews carried out by periodicals such as *Pulse, GP, Practice Computing*, etc. These, and other medical periodicals, regularly carry features comparing systems, and occasionally comment on support and related issues.

Finally, if the supplier of your proposed system is small, you should consider making checks about the financial viability of the company concerned. The trading accounts of limited companies are available for inspection from Companies House in most cases, and a company with few assets and/or little trading profit should normally be avoided unless a satisfactory reason can be found. Similarly, if a company is not registered as a limited company you should seek an explanation.

Deciding on a Specification

Specifications for hardware can be decided in a number of stages. First, decide the number and location of screens. Carefully consider the nature of the tasks that will be performed at them. It is normally necessary to have more than one screen in the reception area in all but the smallest practices, unless reception staff will have easy access to screens in other areas.

If the chosen system uses a network, then each screen will be part of a personal computer (PC), and as such may well also be set up with a general-purpose word processor or spreadsheet. If the system configuration is multi-user then the screens can be dumb terminals, although at the time of writing it is normally better to connect PCs to the system and use software so that they *emulate* a terminal. If PCs are to be used instead of terminals, the specification need not be very high, and a suggested *base* specification is shown in Appendix 3.

Often when a system is ordered, the number of printers is reduced in order to save costs. If screens are installed in consulting rooms then printers should also be installed. A dedicated FP10 repeat prescription printer is always needed in addition to a general-purpose printer to produce letters and reports. Note that on a multi-user system which uses a multiplexer (basically a device which allows several screens and printers to be plugged into the main computer), it is important to allow for some expansion in this unit. An eight-port multiplexer is inadequate in most situations if it has five screens and three printers plugged into it. In this case there would be no economical way of adding further screens and printers without replacing or adding to the multiplexer. A better choice in this situation would be a 12-port unit and larger practices might need up to 60. Similar comments apply to the network hubs which have recently become popular with local-area-network- (LAN)-based systems.

The main computer (or *fileserver*) should be well specified so as to allow for expansions. The specifications of PCs are rapidly changing, but a minimum specification for a file server is shown in Appendix 2. It is of the utmost importance to obtain adequate hard-disk space at the outset, and even the smallest practice should now be considering a hard disk of at least 6 Gb capacity. After only a year many practices have to upgrade their hard-disk units at quite a high cost (owing to engineers visits, etc). A few extra hundred pounds or so at the outset would have avoided the need to do this.

Using Professional Facilitation

In some cases HAs will have general practice facilitators who can help you through the process of choosing a system. Sometimes these facilitators are HA employees and sometimes they are GPs with an interest in computing.

Facilitation can certainly guide you towards the right system for your practice by prompting you to ask the right questions and by considering your proposed usage. Facilitators can normally indicate to you if they have heard of significant problems with a particular system. What facilitators should not do is to decide which system you should have. This is a decision that only the practice staff should make.

Sometimes a GP or a practice manager will ask which is the best system. The reply to this is that there is no such thing and that each general practice system available will have its adherents and its detractors. The *only* way to see if a system will suit your practice is to look at it as carefully and as comprehensively as possible.

There is another good analogy here with cars. Few GPs would expect to be given definite advice on which car would be the best one for them. Instead they would expect to make up their own minds. It is the same with a computer system, the cost of which can be rather more than the average car!

Ordering the System

Once a decision has been made, it is time to place the order for the system.

Make quite sure you fully understand what is, and what is not, included in the system, as already discussed. Try, as far as possible, to make sure that the new system is not delivered at a particularly busy time for the practice. If it is the responsibility of the practice to install the cabling for the system, choose a reliable contractor (ideally one approved by your system supplier) and have all this work completed before the system is delivered. Have a definite plan for implementation of the new system as described in the next chapter. Above all, keep calm!

Closing Summary

> This chapter has attempted to consider some of the important steps which should be taken when a new general practice system is to be purchased. The main points that should be born in mind are:

- *Involve the whole team*
- *Have clear objectives*
- *Define a shortlist*
- *Control system demonstrations*
- *Visit other practices and exhibitions*
- *Look carefully at total costs*
- *Decide hardware layout and specification*
- *Use facilitation, if available*

Chapter 3 considers the commissioning of the system and how its usage might be built up over the first few months.

3
Planning the Initial Use of the General Practice System

Opening Summary

This chapter discusses a methodology for the basic use of the computer system and suggests the order in which different functions can be implemented. Registration, prescribing, cytology and childhood immunisation data is covered, together with some discussion of simple searches.

Introduction

The first six months of use of a new general practice system are often very significant in influencing its long-term use and success. If its implementation is carefully planned and executed, the process of developing system use should be much easier. As at every other stage in the process, it is most important to have a clear idea of what one is trying to achieve.

General Points on Implementation

Many practices implement new clinical computer systems with inadequate thought being given to the intended use of the system, but still manage to use the system effectively. On the other hand, there are many practices where systems have rarely been switched on! Obviously this represents an extreme, but a significant number of practices fall into the following categories:

- Those that master the basics of using their system, but who do not progress beyond this point.
- Those that imput lots of data in an *ad hoc* fashion and hope that it will be converted into useful reports, etc at some (unspecified) time in the future.

Clearly there are many established ways of introducing a new computer system into the practice, but there is no optimum method. To some extent each practice will have to find its own way of working through this process. The important thing is to control the implementation.

The following points should be addressed:

Why?

Why is the system being implemented?

What?

What are the primary objectives? In particular, what are the first steps to be taken? If you have followed the processes suggested in Chapter 2, then some of these question might well have already been answered. If not, now is the time to address them. Later in this chapter, a sequence of events for implementation is suggested. It may well be that practical considerations change this. For example, it may be essential to implement general practice links as one of the first tasks, but a clear idea of the practice's priorities will at least help everyone to move in the right direction.

Who?

Who is going to project manage the new system overall and which member of the team will be responsible for different aspects of implementation? Generally the project manager should be one of the partners or the practice manager, but occasionally the role falls to the computer operator or the practice nurse. All the key players involved in the implementation of a new system should have protected time for their allotted tasks. This is especially important during training sessions. It is often the case during initial training sessions at practices that some participants are called away to deal with day-to-day problems in the practice. This is very disruptive and must be avoided if at all possible.

Where?

Where is each operation going to take place? This again harks back to the planning stage. At this point a decision should be reached as to where each aspect of data entry will take place. For example, in a recently visited practice the nurse was entering smear information on to a computer in reception. A problem arose when the receptionists needed access to this screen for repeat reissues and the arrangement was obviously not working well. Generally data entry should take place either at the location of the initiating event or, in the case of data being entered retrospectively, in some reasonably quiet environment away from the reception area.

When?

When is the best time to implement the new system? The normal answer to this is 'never'. There will be, for the foreseeable future, very great pressures on practices, but it should be borne in mind that in the end a well-implemented system will make the practice more efficient in a variety of ways and will even save time in specific areas!

Notwithstanding the above, there are a variety of situations which make the process of introducing a computer system more difficult, and they should be avoided:

- When moving to new premises.
- When a key member of staff (e.g. the practice manager) is absent for a significant period.
- During some other major change to the practice.
- During or just after a partnership change or split.

The project manager should estimate timescales for each separate stage in the initial implementation of the system. In most cases the timescales will have to be extended. However, the main point of this exercise is that those persons involved will at least be able to measure progress and see how the initial expectations are being fulfilled.

When Should the Practice as a Whole be Introduced to the Use of the System?

Normally receptionists will be introduced to the basics of using the system for registration tasks in the early days of the implementation program. It is sometimes more successful if the GPs do not become too involved at an early stage (unless they are very keen and motivated). The nurses are often the next group of people to start using the system followed by the GPs.

There have been practices where everyone was positively and successfully involved from day one, but these practices are few and far between.

How Should the Practice as a Whole be Introduced to the Use of the System?

The answer to this question has, to a certain extent, been covered in the above four sections, but the main answer is 'gradually'. Many practices are over-ambitious in the first few weeks of the new computer system and then rapidly loose enthusiasm. It is far better to take a slower but realisable approach. One possible scheme for implementation is proposed in Table 3.1. This can be used as a guide, or at least as an example, of a planning document which the practice can produce.

Finally, in case all of the above should look a little daunting, remember that suppliers have considerable experience of helping practices in the initial stages of using their new computer systems.

Strategies and Practical Issues

All practices will have existing information systems either in computer databases or in manual form. Clearly, it is important to consider how this data will be entered into the new clinical system. We will consider first the general points of transferring manual data.

During the initial stages it is most important that all members of the team are involved in the process. Problems occur when individuals independently develop their usage in ways that make it difficult to achieve consistency and completeness of data entry.

Manual Data Entry

Many practices, especially those that have not been computerised before, will have manually recorded data. It is important to enter this data into the computer as soon as possible. Examples include cytology or immunisation data recorded in a ledger or on a card-index-based system.

Clearly, the two above examples are different in the sense that there is likely to be more cytology records to deal with than childhood immunisation data. In the case of the latter it would be possible for one person to enter the data on to the computer in just a few weeks – if they were given protected time to do this.

In the case of cytology (and assuming that there is no alternative source of electronic data, i.e. the HA) the task is likely to take rather longer. However, even in the largest practices the task should be possible in several weeks rather than in several months.

Often data of the above type is entered but the method by which the data is searched is not considered. The syndrome is 'we'll sort out how to do the searches later because we don't have time at present'. Clearly, this can lead to a lot of trouble later. I make no apology for stressing this several times, as the whole basis of the use of a general practice computer system can fail on this one point.

Table 3.1 One possible scheme for the implementation of basic functions

Task	Who	When
Registration data *by* HA download *or* conversion of old data	Supplier	Before/at delivery
Checking registration data	Practice manager and/or computer operator and/or receptionists	As soon as possible (0–8 weeks)
Testing/running registration searches	Practice manager and/or computer operator	As soon as possible (0–8 weeks)
Start using/maintaining registration data	Practice manager and/or computer operator and/or receptionists	> 8 weeks
Links–registration*	Practice manager Computer operator HA/supplier	As appropriate – might be the first task in some cases
Repeat prescribing data by manual entry and/or conversion of old data	Practice manager Computer operator Receptionists Supplier	8–16 weeks
Implement repeat prescribing system	All (including GPs, if possible)	> 17 weeks
Cytology data by manual entry or conversion of old data	Practice manager and/or computer operator and/or nurse	24–30 weeks (if manually entering data)
Test cytology reports	Practice manager and/or computer operator and/or nurse	24–30 weeks
Implement cytology	Practice manager and/or computer operator and/or nurse	> 30 weeks
Childhood immunisation data by manual entry or conversion of old data	Practice manager and/or computer operator and/or nurse	24–30 weeks (if manually entering data)
Test child immunisation reports	Practice manager and/or computer operator and/or nurse	24–30 weeks
Implement cytology and child immunisations	Practice manager and/or computer operator and/or nurse	> 30 weeks

*Links normally also includes a list matching phase which is covered more fully in Chapter 10

There are two main methods by which a large amount of manually held patient data can be installed on to a computer:

- Opportunistically.
- Sequentially

Each has advantages and disadvantages. Opportunistic data entry is probably easier for the practice to accommodate. It implies entering the data on to the computer when a patient's manual records are accessed, e.g. prior to a surgery visit. Data entry by this method can take a long time to complete and a few patients may never be added. However, it is less tedious than any type of sequential approach. Using sequential entry the practice starts with the A's and progresses slowly to the Z's. The biggest problem of this approach is that the Z's are not always reached, as the task is just too enormous. The advantage is that, in theory, no patient will be excluded.

Electronic Data Entry

Data transfer via electronic methods brings its own problems. These can be summarised as

- Is it accurate?
- Is it in the correct location?

Data that is grossly inaccurate can take almost as long to correct as to enter from scratch. Data coming from any external source is unlikely to be 100% accurate and up to date. Practices should carefully consider the implications of inaccurate data. It is likely that any software supplier converting data will have a disclaimer from the partners absolving the supplier of all responsibility for the accuracy of the data. It is nearly always the case that some data is lost when converting from one system to another.

Data should also be loaded in any new system *into its correct location*. It is of little use to load, for example, coded clinical data as free text. As Read codes become more widely used for all aspects of patient records, the process of transferring data should become easier.

We will now consider specific types of data.

Registration Data

Most practices embarking on their first clinical system will have a *Health Authority Download* of registration data for their patients. This data will originate from the HA computer system and will be supplied to the system supplier, who will then pre-load the information on to the system. In the past the quality of this information has often been somewhat at variance with manual registration data held by the

Planning the Initial Use of the General Practice System 45

practice. Generally, nowadays, the quality of the data is much better although it may be lacking in scope. Although the basic data of fields such as name, address, DOB, etc may be accurate, it may lack other details which the practice wishes to record, e.g. telephone number or next of kin.

Despite the fact that the data will mostly be correct, it may still be necessary to check the data to ensure its accuracy.

Nowadays almost all practices that are computerising for the first time will also be implementing *general practice registration links*. In this situation a download from the HA could be a positive advantage as the exact format of the name and address fields will be the same at both the HA and the practice. This obviates the need for any list-matching process to be undertaken. In the event of practice registration data being transferred from a previous computer system, there should be few, if any, problems. It is possible, however, that the new computer system may not have a field or 'slot' for the data to go into easily, and the registration status of a significant number of patients will change during the transfer to the new system. However, if general practice links are to be used the data will have to be list-matched. This will involve comparing the HA and practice records for each patient and correcting minor typographical details such as spaces and capitalisation. Links will be considered in more detail in Chapter 9.

In many cases the practice will wish to record more registration information in the 'new' computer system than was possible in the 'old' system. The motivation for this is often that more registration fields exist and so the practice feels under a certain pressure to fill them in.

As is always the case, there should be clear reasons for entering data into the registration screen and the information entered should:

- Be useful in respect of that specific patient.
- Be useful in terms of data extraction.

As an example, a field for mileage units for a patient is most useful with respect to claims *for that patient* and it is unlikely (although not impossible) that the practice would want to run searches on this data. On the other hand, a field for registration category, although important on an individual basis, is also data that the practice is likely to wish to search, e.g. so as to extract all active patients.

Finally, as already mentioned, practices often spend far too little time working out how they are going to use the computer effectively to improve the efficiency of the practice. It is essential to work out fully how the registration data is going to be searched and reported in order to prevent the practice from having to search manual records. The completion of the various registration forms required by the HA should be facilitated by the use of the computer for registration. It should not be a pointless extra task.

The following example is typical:

> ... We've had the computer for six months now and we are getting on quite well. We always register new patients on the computer but we have not been shown how to do registration searches. We have to use the old manual system in order to find all the changes of registration status for the HA. Also with our system we can't find a way to show that a patient is a temporary resident for more than 15 days so we register the patient for GMS and then put a comment in the 'any other information' field at the end of the registration screen. We had not been told that we shouldn't have indicated a temporary resident in this way and we can't search for temporary residents now until we ...

Once the practice had been shown how to enter the data properly *and* how to do registration searches, the problem diminished. The main point is that if they had clarified the searching and the entry of temporary residents *before* embarking on data entry, they could have prevented a lot of extra work.

Prescribing

Once the registration aspects of a system have been clarified, the next logical area of the new computer system to implement is prescribing. The question here is 'Should the practice attempt all the prescribing on the computer or should only repeats be tackled – at least in the first instance?' The main difference between prescribing and registration data is that GPs can have a significant involvement in prescribing.

As with all other aspects of system use, there are advantages and disadvantages to each approach, and practices must find a level of progress which suits them. It is to be hoped that long before they actually acquire their new computer system they will have decided on the way in which they wish to develop. However, this may have to be modified in the light of experience once the system is up and running. Below are some of the points that should be addressed, together with some comments on them:

> *1. Does the practice possess the hardware to make prescribing by GPs a practical proposition? In particular, does each GP have a suitable printer for acutes or can they easily access an FP10 printer elsewhere? In the latter case how does the prescription reach the patient?*

In a practice where individual GPs do not have terminals on their desk, prescribing by GPs is clearly not a practical proposition. In many practices some of the GPs have a terminal in their rooms while those who are less interested do not. In this mixed situation it is questionable as to whether any general practice based prescribing is a worthwhile enterprise, as the practice will, in any case, have to accommodate those GPs who are not equipped with a computer.

If GPs wish to use the system to issue acute prescriptions then it is almost essential for them also to have a printer in their consulting room. Although in theory various ways of circumventing this can be devised, these options seldom work well in practice.

2. Do the majority of the GPs have the resolve to initiate repeat/and acute prescribing in the consultation?

Clearly, if some GPs in the practice are not convinced of the benefits of using the computer for prescribing they will not do it. It is often the case, particularly in relation to repeats, that GPs are fully convinced of the benefits provided they do not personally have to set up the scripts. Some GPs are often less enthusiastic regarding the benefits of acute prescribing and, as has already been mentioned, the most persuasive of these is the goal of a complete searchable prescribing record for the practice as well as every individual patient.

3. Is the system sufficiently user friendly for the process to be practicable?

It is in the nature of general practice that most GPs are extremely busy and are also faced with constantly having to assimilate new information on developments in treatments, etc. Few have the time to learn complicated sets of non-intuitive keystrokes. Although the ease of prescribing should have been carefully reviewed at the time the system was selected, this area is easy to overlook.

4. Do all the GPs know how to use the prescribing features and, if not, who is going to help them learn?

If a system is difficult or time consuming to use in this respect, it is very important to set up a training session and take all the potential users through the easiest method of achieving the desired result. Single page guides are useful not only for new users but also for any temporary practice members, such as locums.

5. Will the practice try to enforce a policy of generic prescribing, and, if so, how will the system help in this respect? Is a practice formulary in operation, and, if so, how can this be implemented on the computer?

Different computer systems have many different ways of helping the practice to prescribe generically. The systems range from those that have absolutely no features to those that provide a variety of measures.

These include:

- Systems that allow the setting up of a practice formulary as an alternative to the full drug database.
- Systems that learn which drug forms are most often used and place these choices at the top of picking lists.
- Systems that allow the selection of the generic form of a drug by pressing a key when the non-generic form of the drug has been selected.

Even in the case of systems that have no specific features to help in this respect, it is possible for the practice to agree a finite list of common drug forms that will be used. With these systems it is also often possible to edit the drug file directly and remove non-preferred forms of drugs, if desired.

6. Are there any shortcuts that can be used to speed up the process of prescribing? Are there various ways into the prescribing module, and which, if any, is the preferred route?

Many current systems allow the user to set up a programmed series of keystrokes which can be 'played back' by pressing a key combination. Sometimes such features are a function of the terminals in use and sometimes they are a feature of the software. Many practices find such features very useful and 'record' all the most common drugs (in their most common forms) so that they can be accessed and issued in this way. One name for this type of feature is *macro* and the process is sometimes termed *playing back a macro*. This feature, which also goes under several other names, can be a useful time-saver for those GPs who are not used to using a keyboard as well as for ensuring consistency. The potential downside is that the key combination might be pressed accidentally, and hence a drug might be issued for a patient unintentionally, and then be recorded. This can normally be avoided by using unusual key combinations such as F10-f-z or Alt-6.

In terms of implementing prescribing on the computer, it was said previously that practices should find a speed of implementation which suits them. Some GPs will attempt to put all prescribing on to the computer from day one. Often this approach fails in much the same way as over-enthusiastic dieting cannot be sustained. It is normally better to approach the issue gradually and build up data input in prescribing (or any other area) over a period of months. In this way surgery times are not grossly lengthened and keyboard skills improve as more data is gradually entered.

Cytology and Immunisations

Cytology screening and childhood immunisations are probably the next areas that a practice would normally wish to implement.

Both these topics involve recording data using either Read codes or some other system. This data is then searched, normally using pre-written search routines, to see if the targets have been reached and/or which individuals need to be targeted.

Many of the points relevant to registration are also relevant here. In particular it is vital to make sure that the search routines work as expected. If they do not appear to work then it may be that data is not being entered in the correct way.

If data has been transferred from another system it is possible that some elements of the data may not translate properly to the new system. This is probably more likely if the original system was one where the data was not Read coded and the 'new' system does have Read codes. In any case, it is important that it is systematically checked.

Clearly, the accuracy of the data is essential – there is little point in a computerised screening system which does not fulfil its purpose. Practices carrying out searches for the first time often have difficulty in selecting qualifying ages and date ranges for reports.

Simple Predefined Searches

Suppliers of medical systems normally provide a variety of predefined searches as well as a report generator for more complex searches.

Some of the most common predefined searches are those which cover such essential topics as cytology, immunisation targets and basic health data. The number and scope of such searches varies widely from supplier to supplier. The basic approach to such searches also varies. Normally they would either be

- Simple saved searches of the type which can be produced with the system report generator, *or*
- Totally different in format and scope to the reports which the user can produce in the report generator.

It does not matter much which type of report is used, although fully custom-written reports can be more tailored to a particular task than can the former. It is important to note that some suppliers use the word 'report' to refer to the whole process of searching for patients and printing the results. Others split the process into two distinct stages: firstly, the *search* to isolate the particular group of patients, and secondly the *report* that specifies which details of these patients will be printed.

A general principle that applies to all searches is that of GIGO. This is an acronym for 'garbage in garbage out'. This long-standing expression implies that searches are only as good as the data that has been entered, and hence if data is incomplete or inaccurate, then obviously so is the report.

For this reason stress should be placed on understanding how the standard reports work at an early stage in the development of the system and also that all data entered is validated.

Notwithstanding the above, things can and do go wrong.

> A small practice in east London had been using a well-known general practice system from one of the largest suppliers for about nine months. They had embarked on an ambitious and widespread program of data entry and now they wanted to be able to search for the data and produce some reports. The computer system in question is powerful and flexible *but only searches by Read code*. These GPs had arranged for all of the data to be entered into free text, even to the extent of test results and common values such as BPs. The net result was that it was impossible to extract any data from the system at this stage.

> At another practice, the staff were surprised to find that when they ran a search for the number of asthmatics in the practice the number picked up was much smaller that expected. On looking at the entered data the reason for this was self-evident. There were two data entry clerks at the practice – the GPs were not entering data – and one had identified asthmatics with the code 'H/O Asthma' meaning 'history of asthma', whereas the other had been using the code 'Asthma', which falls in an entirely different part of the Read classification.
>
> As the search had only been carried out on one of these codes, all those patients with the other code were not found.

In some instances when searches are run it is obvious that the results are incorrect, but this is not always the case. Often there is a danger that a neat printed report will be 'believed', even though the data is inaccurate. Most people seem to have an in-built predisposition to believe reports that are generated from a computer, whereas in fact it may be better to maintain a healthy scepticism.

Closing Summary

It is essential to plan which items of data are going to be entered on the computer in the first instance. The personnel involved in the data entry should be clearly identified, as should the precise reasons for the data entry. Methods of searching should be attempted at an early stage to ensure that the intended results can be achieved. Timescales should be realistic but short enough to maintain the impetus for achieving a particular goal. Those practice members involved in the implementation of the system should have protected time to complete this work. Data transferred to a new system by electronic methods from an old system should be carefully checked for accuracy.

Time spent in planning the initial implementation of the system will be repaid in more efficient (and ultimately more widespread) use of the system.

4
Further Uses of the General Practice System

Opening Summary

This chapter deals with some of the more advanced uses of the clinical system that might be implemented after the basic uses have been mastered. Specifically, the writing of recall letters and the entry of clinical data are covered.

General Points

Chapter 3 dealt with the first uses made of the clinical computer system. This chapter looks at some of the areas that should come next in the planned implementation of the system.

In many cases the new computer system will have caused significant disruption and extra workload for members of the practice team, and the last thing that anybody wants to think about is further changes to existing working practices. In this case is it often better to wait awhile before bringing new aspects of the system in to use rather, than implementing things in a piecemeal fashion. In all cases it is important to convince the whole practice team (or at least most members of it) that the new uses are worthwhile.

Whereas there is little point in trying to force the pace of change, a too relaxed approach can be less than useful. Many practices, while they have mastered the basic uses of their system, have not moved on to such things as clinical data entry even over a period of some years. The previous paragraph notwithstanding, it would generally be better to have reached the point where most planned/envisaged system functions are implemented within 18–24 months of first acquiring the system.

The other major danger, if a planned approach to data handling is not adopted, is that certain types of data entry may start to take place in an *ad hoc* and ineffective fashion, as mentioned previously. As ever, the development of the system should be 'sold' on results. The next-month syndrome – 'we really must get round a table and decide how we are going to do this, but not this month, as we have *x/y/z* happening' – must be avoided.

Much stress has been laid on the planning of data entry and *ensuring that data entry will produce the desired result*. If anything, this becomes more important as more advanced data entry is considered. In the case of registration data, cytology and immunisations, it is likely that the number of ways of entering the data will be limited. This is not the case with diseases or symptoms that can often be entered in a number of different ways, depending on the system in question. Always decide precisely what is the purpose of the data entry and test that data can be extracted as expected.

In order to be able to test data entry, it is often a good idea to have a dummy patient on the system with an unusual registration status, e.g. 'private patient' (so as to avoid the patient being picked up by registration links) and an unusual age, e.g. 115 years, so that searches can be isolated to pick up a particular aspect of the record for patients of age > 114. Recently, some suppliers have actually added a registration category of 'fictitious' (or equivalent) so as to facilitate this on a linked system.

More advanced aspects of use are considered in the following sections.

Recall Letters

A recall letter facility allows practices to send personalised letters to just about any group of patients in the practice. Traditionally, it has been used to send out reminder letters for smears and childhood immunisations. In many areas these functions are now taken care of by regional schemes or the HA, and so although the system can be used for the above, more likely uses include the recall of patients for particular clinics or perhaps for a medication change.

The main advantage of using a practice computer system to send out recall and similar letters is that information specific to that patient can be taken from the system where it already resides. The main disadvantage can be that the process of setting up the system can be so complex as to defeat even the most dedicated enthusiast.

In some cases there is an alternative. This is to export the name/address data for the required group of patients from the computer and use it in conjunction with the mail merge facilities of a mainstream word processor package such as Microsoft Word or Corel WordPerfect.

Generally there are three stages in creating a set of recall letters using a clinical system:

1. Decide on how you are going to isolate the target group – normally by carrying out some form of search.
2. Construct a *template* letter in which personalised information in the letter, e.g. name, address, etc is replaced by codes represent-

ing this information generically.
3. Merge the information from the database with the information and layout in the letter so as to produce a number of personalised letters. It may seem complicated, but in a well-designed general practice system it is actually quite straightforward.

As mentioned earlier, in some cases the merge could be carried out using a commercial word processor. The main barrier to this approach is the lack of suitable export facilities in quite a lot of systems so as to produce the *data file* for the commercial system to use.

Occasionally practices find themselves in a situation where the clinical system has neither good merge facilities nor export facilities to extract the data. In this situation it may be worth considering actually rekeying patient address data into a PC to gain access to competent mailmerge facilities. It would still, in most cases, be quicker than resorting to photocopying a standard letter and hand writing in all the details – particularly in those cases where the same group of patients are to be contacted more than once.

Patient Information

This is probably the area where there is the most variation in the information that is entered into the computer. As mentioned in Chapter 2, there are many levels at which patient-encounter information can be tackled:

- Comprehensive data entry.
- Major events only.
- Selected health data entry only.

Like most things, general practice data entry is evolutionary and the limited data entry can often lead gradually to full entry of clinical data. Nowadays whichever route is adopted it is likely to involve the use of Read codes and it is appropriate to develop the material covered in Chapter 2.

Irrespective of the planned final level of data entry, a majority of practices would like to have some consultation data on the computer. At its most basic this could be just that a consultation has taken place, but many would like to have a coded reason for the event. This could be a diagnosis if this is clear, but could equally be a symptom. Finding the appropriate Read code can be time consuming for all but the most common systems.

In the first few months a preferred Read code list can often be most useful both in ensuring that some consistency of coding is adhered to (i.e. 'Asthma' rather than 'History of Asthma' to indicate an asthmatic) and in order to save time. If a common Read code list is in use it is normally possible to enter a specific Read code directly rather than via one of its rubrics – this is normally much quicker. Some systems allow the use of a Read code formulary rather like a drug formulary.

Implementing a Preferred Read Code List

At one time or another many practices have attempted to bring consistency into the Read codes that they use, often with only limited success.

The following method seems to work well. First all the partners in a practice agree to spend a few weeks in opportunistically gathering items which they wish to Read code. They do this by assessing each patient they see in their surgeries and applying the following criteria:

- Is the symptom that the patient describes a symptom on which we might wish to carry out a search?
- Is the disease that the patient is suffering from a disease group that we wish to be able to identify?

If neither of the above is true, do I still have a good reason for Read coding this event/symptom/disease? For example, would it be quicker to enter a Read code rather than a textual description?

If the answer to the first question is 'yes' then the GP writes down the symptom on a piece of paper. At this point he/she does not bother to try and find the appropriate Read code. Likewise, if the answer to the second question is 'yes', the appropriate disease is written down. Finally, if the item qualifies by virtue of the third question, it is recorded.

After a couple of weeks each GP will have a list with a fairly extensive range of items on it. In some cases the GPs may have encountered the same symptom or disease several times, in which case they should simply indicate this by putting a tick (or ticks) against the entry.

The list might look something like that shown below:

```
Essential hypertension      ✓✓✓✓✓
Asthma                      ✓✓
D&V                         ✓✓
Bleeding from bowel         ✓✓✓
Low back pain               ✓
etc, etc
```

At a regular practice meeting the GPs take it in turn to read out items from their individual lists. If different GPs have used different words to describe essentially the same thing, they agree on a common form. The entry – provided all agree it qualifies – is transferred to a master list (still not Read coded) and the next GP takes his turn. This process should not be carried out all at once, but a little at a time, until one agreed list of proposed items exists. At this stage the size of the list indicates (empirically) the long-term success of the scheme such that:

- *List of 50 or less items:* A good chance of successful implementation.
- *List 50–100 items:* A reasonable chance of successful implementation.
- *List 100–150 items:* A fair chance if the entire practice staff are strongly committed to the process.
- *List 150+ items:* Increasingly less chance of success as the list size increases.

Having arrived at a common list of items, these can then be matched to Read codes so as to produce the desired Read code list. In doing this matching it would be well to choose a code or codes carefully *from the appropriate part of the Read hierarchy*. This list can then be wordprocessed and arranged so that the GPs can enter the appropriate code, either by typing in some of the rubric, or the actual alpha-numeric code, as desired.

Some systems will allow the setting up of internal picking lists based on just these codes.

An example of part of a typical list is shown in Table 4.1. Note that the list has been arranged by body system rather than alphabetically, as this would seem to be the most efficient order for GPs to use easily.

Table 4.1 Portion of typical Read code list

Term	Code	Term	Code
Cardiovascular		Gastroenterology	
angina pectoris	G33	acute appendicitis	J120
aortic aneurysm	G71	appendicectomy	7701z
atrial fibrillation	G5730	cancer of gut	B1...
congenital heart disease	P5	cholecystectomy	7810
congestive heart failure	G580	coeliac disease	J690
coronary artery surgery	792	colostomy	771B
etc	etc	etc	etc

Having created a list for initial use, it is best just to get on and use it, making modifications where necessary. One danger is that if too much time is spent creating the perfect list the job is never actually finished. If all clinical members of the team then use the list, in about 12–18 months the practice will have the ability to extract useful data from the system. The idea of a list is not meant to be restrictive, but instead to form a *minimum* standard. There is nothing to stop those who wish to do so coding additional items or using Read codes to greater levels of accuracy, although there should be clear reasons for doing this.

At this point it is appropriate to cover the other main type of data that is often entered into computer systems, i.e. numeric data. This covers a wide range of items, from basic ones such as height and weight to items such as blood glucose levels, FBCs, etc.

Quite a lot of the numeric data that can be stored on a clinical system comes from laboratory tests, and nowadays the easiest way to input this data on to the system is via an electronic link to the laboratory. Some suppliers are not yet offering this facility, and, in other cases, the laboratories in question are not set up to deal with the electronic delivery of information.

In either of these cases the only approach is to enter the data by hand, but the benefits of this must be clearly identifiable, as the workload involved for the practice can be considerable. It is also worth checking that numeric data can be adequately searched as, at the time of writing, systems still exist which allow the entry of numeric data but which offer little or no facilities for searching it.

Comprehensive Data Entry

Many GPs feel that this would be fine in an ideal world, but raise various objections in practice – particularly the time it takes. Further, many GPs feel legally and/or practically obliged to keep manual records for the foreseeable future and cannot justify keeping two sets of records. Some cannot see much general advantage in the approach, but this is often a function of the particular system in use.

The main advantages of fully computerised medical records are 'structure' and accessibility to the data. What is meant by 'structure' is that it is possible to examine data in the records in ways that would not be possible in conventional manual records. For example, it should be possible in a well-designed system to look at a particular 'problem' and at all of the consultations, prescribing and other details of it in isolation from the rest of the record. Even in the most well-organised manual records this would normally be difficult.

Accessibility covers a variety of things including:

- The ability to be able to carry out complex searches so as to isolate groups of patients or to do an audit.
- Access to a full patient record from all parts of the surgery that have screens, and also sometimes from home.
- More physical security, in that if the computer is destroyed or stolen, it is easy to recreate the records from the backup.
- More physical security in that even if unauthorised persons gain

access to the computer they are unlikely to be able to gain access to patient records without a password.

There are many data aspects involved in the above, not only consultation data, but also significant amounts of medical history needs to be entered, ideally as well as test requests and results, and referral letters and their responses from secondary care. Few practices succeed in getting all this information on to the computer at once – the important thing, as ever, is to plan carefully.

Major Events Only

In this situation the practice makes a policy decision not to attempt to enter all patient encounters and other data on to the computer, but rather to concentrate on significant items only plus basic health data. Clearly there are many different ways of interpreting this situation, but as an example, the practice might, in addition to basic health data, decide to record only 'major events' for their patients on the computer. One definition of a major event would be to enter items such as those that would be recorded on a summary card in the manual notes.

This approach leads to some, but not all, of the advantages mentioned in the previous section and is often adopted as a forerunner to a more comprehensive policy. In particular, it allows:

- Searches to isolate groups of patients or to do audit, although it is likely that there would be insufficient data for sophisticated audits.
- Access to a basic patient record from all parts of the surgery with screens such that, in the absence of the manual records, at least the most important patient data is available.
- Some physical security, in that if the computer is destroyed or stolen, it is easy to recreate a basic record from the backup

Selected Health Data Entry Only

Many practices adopt this policy. As a first step on the way to the successful use of the computer system it is a good approach. Even with basic data such as this there are many things that can go wrong, but as always it pays both to be consistent and to check that required searches can be done, before entering too much data.

The main emphasis of this kind of data entry is to enter information needed for essential reporting activities. Items such as heights, weights, family history information, smoking habits, BP, etc is typical of this type of data.

How Should Clinical Data be Entered?

Implementing the above is a major step forward on the route to the electronic clinical record and multiple disease registers. Another major factor is, having decided what data needs to be entered, deciding where to enter it. Some of the major systems (i.e. EMIS, AAH Meditel) allow searches to be carried out irrespective of where the data was entered, but some of the smaller systems have separate areas (i.e. consultations and medical history, etc) and these areas can only be searched individually. Although a major system, VAMP Medical will currently allow family history information to be entered into history as an *OXMIS* code or as a line in a *Freehand* screen. The two are not connected, and, as a result, if some data has been entered into both a search for all the information can be overly complex.

This really comes back to the principals, which have already been mentioned, namely

- *Be aware of the purpose of data entry.*
- *Make sure that the data entry used can produce the desired outputs.*

If you do use a system which has multiple unlinked data-entry areas, decide *where* certain types of data will be stored. This is nearly as important a point as *what* to store.

When we discussed the benefits of computer systems as well as the benefits accruing from being able to extract bulk data, the idea of the structured electronic record was mentioned. Some general practice systems have a more structured record than others, but this is really the ability to present the data in a variety of different ways. But what is a structured record and how is it superior to paper records?

Structured Electronic Records

EMIS, AAH Meditel and, more recently, VAMP Vision, are probably the best examples of systems with structured clinical records.

In a structured record it is possible to look at the data in a variety of ways, provided it has been entered correctly in the first place. Different systems implement this in slightly different ways, but with these systems at the very least it is possible to look at a particular problem and then see details of all the consultations relating to the problem, including the medication issued in response to it.

As an example, if a particular patient comes to their GP complaining of burning pains in the stomach then a new problem (Read coded) such as dyspepsia (J16y4) might be created. Linked to this, the GP might record some free text and also any medication issued.

Later, if the patient returns for a further consultation relating to the same problem, the second consultation with its details can be linked to the first. In this way, if a period of time elapses and then patients come to see their GPs about pre-existing conditions, it is easy for them to look quickly at the data related to the problems. Otherwise they might have to trawl through the manual notes or pick items out from a larger list on the computer. If the problem on diagnosis is clarified, then the title can be changed, but all of the note entries retained, as before.

Of course, even if a computer offers a structured record or a problem-oriented approach, it is only useful it this approach is used by all those concerned with clinical data entry. Many practices have systems which are capable of storing data in this way, but are not used to do so. Instead every new encounter is recorded as a new problem, removing some of the benefits of the system.

Templates

A *template* is defined as a form presented on screen for the entry of data. Templates are screen forms; they present a number of related data items together to make data entry quicker. For example, if a practice wishes to monitor their diabetic patients, it would be possible at each clinic attendance or consultation to enter each item separately on to the computer. So, assuming that some of the items of interest would be BP, Ht, Wt, fundi check OK, etc it would mean finding the appropriate code and entering data four times (in a real situation a diabetic template could easily contain 20–30 data items). A diabetic template presents prompts for these items and they can simply be filled in.

The use of templates should lead to the following benefits:

- Consistency
- Speed of data entry
- Completeness of data

Figure 4 shows a template (Freehand Screen) from a VAMP Medical system.

Templates are important tools in the entry of data for chronic disease management and as such are most likely to be used extensively by nurses. They are also useful in consultation situations where a number of *related* data items need to be input. They can also be used to enter previously collated data or to identify missing data. One of the main reasons why GPs are reluctant to use them is that a lot of templates have been designed to be used by nurses and are too long for regular GP use. A solution to this might be to have a number of templates for each condition, such as for diabetes. Of these, one might be for the initial encounter, one for repeat encounters and one for GP use in consultations. The one for GPs would be likely to be much shorter than the others, and would only cover those data items that would be relevant in this situation.

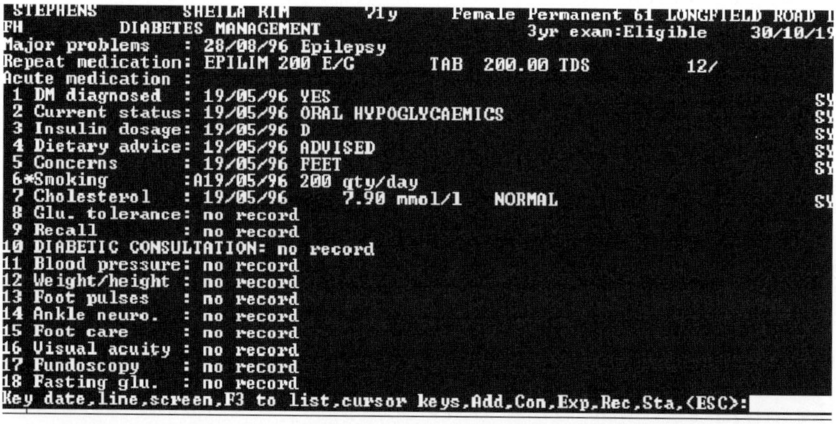

```
STEPHENS          SHEILA KIM         71y      Female Permanent 61 LONGFIELD ROAD
PH          DIABETES MANAGEMENT                3yr exam:Eligible    30/10/19
Major problems    : 28/08/96 Epilepsy
Repeat medication: EPILIM 200 E/C          TAB  200.00 TDS        12/
Acute medication :
 1 DM diagnosed   : 19/05/96 YES                                              SY
 2 Current status : 19/05/96 ORAL HYPOGLYCAEMICS                              SY
 3 Insulin dosage : 19/05/96 D                                                SY
 4 Dietary advice : 19/05/96 ADVISED                                          SY
 5 Concerns       : 19/05/96 FEET                                             SY
 6*Smoking        :A19/05/96 200 qty/day
 7 Cholesterol    : 19/05/96     7.90 mmol/l    NORMAL                        SY
 8 Glu. tolerance : no record
 9 Recall         : no record
10 DIABETIC CONSULTATION= no record
11 Blood pressure : no record
12 Weight/height  : no record
13 Foot pulses    : no record
14 Ankle neuro.   : no record
15 Foot care      : no record
16 Visual acuity  : no record
17 Fundoscopy     : no record
18 Fasting glu.   : no record
Key date,line,screen,F3 to list,cursor keys,Add,Con,Exp,Rec,Sta,<ESC>:
```

Figure 4   The VAMP Medical freehand template screen

Earlier in this chapter it was mentioned that users should be aware of whether or not data entered in one part of a system is accessible in other areas. In the case of templates in particular, it is important to know if:

- The data is held in templates separately from the other data.
- The data form part of problems.
- The data collected by the template is Read coded.
- The format of the template can be changed.

This last point is very important, as a number of systems supply templates but do not allow the users to modify them. Although these templates are still useful, in most cases it is much better if the practice staff can modify templates themselves.

In cases where the clinical system allows templates to be modified, this is sometimes too technical a task for the practice concerned (e.g. SOPHIE in AAH Meditel is a very powerful template and protocol system, but can be difficult to use in design mode). In this case, there are often other ways to obtain alternative templates and a good source is often the user group for the system concerned. It is still a good idea for at least one person in each practice to gain the essential skills to be able to change existing templates and, if necessary, to be able to create a new one from scratch.

One of the differences between data entered in templates and data entered more generally is that in the former case it is possible for an individual to take charge of a certain area reasonably easily. For example, a nurse who is looking after asthmatics in a practice can fill in data in the template for all the patients in this group reasonably quickly, and can start to output data in specific audits. This is in contrast to unstructured methods of data entry that involve other members of the practice, where it can take some time to identify the data needed for reports.

Before leaving the subject of templates, it is important to distinguish between templates and protocols. This is because the terms are in use in a loosely interchangeable way in primary care, but there are important differences between them. Perhaps the easiest way to distinguish between them is to say that

- **A template** *is a form presented on screen for the entry of data.*
- **A protocol**, *although somewhat similar, is able to follow preset rules, and as such respond to data entered, so that further data items are appropriate. In other words, depending on a response, it can branch to a different area and ask different questions.*

For example, a peak flow reading entered into a template will simply become a piece of stored data – abnormal values might cause a warning to be displayed, but otherwise the template merely goes on to the next item.

A protocol, on the other hand, might *respond* to the value in a number of ways:

- A normal value might make it simply move on the next item of data – rather like the template.
- A mildly abnormal value might change the next prompt and/or have an effect on suggested medication.
- A grossly abnormal value might terminate the protocol with a warning that the patient should be referred to a GP immediately.

In other words, the protocol has the ability to go off down different paths depending on the responses given. This makes it both more powerful than a normal template and considerably more difficult to set up, and most practices should become thoroughly used to the idea of using templates prior to moving on to protocols (in systems where these are available).

Searches, Audits and Reports

Simple predefined searches have already been covered in an earlier section and it is now appropriate to discuss more complex searches that might be set up by the practice.

There are many reasons why practices might wish to run their own searches. These would include:

- Information needed by the practice to claim income.
- Audits.
- Information needed in response to a drug recall.
- Information needed for the practice's annual report.

Clearly, there are many different methods of searching clinical systems depending on the system concerned, but certain general principles can be covered here.

Indexes

A few clinical systems offer the choice of indexed or non-indexed searches, or, in some cases, a combination of both. Often the only easy way to distinguish an indexed search from a non-indexed search is that the former runs at about ten times the speed of the latter.

To understand indexes, consider a thick reference book. At the back is an alphabetical index of the topics of the book and the page numbers on which they occur. To find a certain topic you can do one of two things:

1. Start at page one and scan every page until you find the desired topic.
2. Look up the topic in the index, and then proceed straight away to the relevant page.

The second approach is clearly much faster, and this is why indexed searches are much faster on a computer. Of course, the difference between a book and a computer is that the book will normally only have one alphabetical index whereas the computer can have an index on virtually any field or combination of fields. This leads us to the question 'Why not index every field to make all searches fast?'. The problem here is that although this would indeed make searches very fast, it would slow down the computer during normal use as it went through the work of creating or updating large numbers of indexes.

As an example of the relevance of the above, consider a search for women with asthma on an AAH Meditel system. With this system you can combine an indexed and a non-indexed search in one operation. If you were looking for female asthmatics in AAH Meditel you could first find all the women (using an index), then look through these records sequentially to isolate the asthmatics. Alternatively, you could use an index to isolate all asthmatics (via the Read codes) and then look through these records sequentially to find those who were female. In this example the second approach would be a lot quicker. In contrast, using EMIS the exact method of selection is unimportant owing to a much greater reliance on the use of indexed searches in this system.

ANDs, ORs and NOTs

In many situations, searching involves looking for patient records based on a number of conditions. For instance, patients who are *both* diabetic and asthmatic might need to be searched for and identified. This search contains an 'AND'. This implies that records will only be selected from the search if *both* asthma *and* diabetes are present, using the appropriate method – normally Read codes – to identify them. Implicitly in the above, patients with asthma alone or diabetes alone will be excluded. In order to identify patients who are *either* asthmatic *or* diabetic, you would search for either asthmatics *or* diabetics.

On some systems you can use a 'NOT' operator as well. This means that you can search for asthmatics that are not diabetic or vice versa. The three terms AND, OR and NOT are technically known as Boolean operators and it is important to understand how your system handles these concepts. The only thing worse than not being able to do a search, is unintentionally doing the wrong one and consequently ending up answering a question that you did not ask.

Read Codes and Searching

Most of the issues regarding Read codes have been covered earlier, but it is true to say that practices often have lots of problems in undertaking specific searches. To illustrate these, consider a search for females who are pregnant.

If the practice searches for women who have a Read code (or some other code) for pregnancy then a large proportion of the practice population will appear in the search. If a data range is then applied, what date range do you use? If the last nine months is used, there will still be problems owing to terminations, miscarriages, etc. One way to handle the above is use the term 'pregnant' to indicate *currently pregnant* and to replace it with another code after a birth. This is all right but implies removing information from the patient record, which is generally undesirable.

As another example, consider a diabetic classified as NIDDM who then becomes IDDM. Searches for IDDM and NIDDM patients will both include this patient unless the previous status is removed – not a good idea – or a more complex search is carried out. One solution to the above is to search for NIDDMs who do *not* have an IDDM code.

There are many examples of the above and, as ever, it comes down to carefully planning what you are trying to achieve. *Always think about the result BEFORE embarking on data entry.*

Another point to bear in mind is always to be aware of how your Read codes are being selected. Virtually all Read-coded systems allow the user to search either for a specific Read code or from a Read code to the bottom of the hierarchy. Make sure that it is clearly understood which is being done, or else there will be unexpected results.

Finally, as already mentioned many times before, plan data entry carefully. It is inconvenient to search for a condition if no system has been applied to the data entry and the condition has been loosely entered under a number of Read hierarchies.

Export to PCs for Further Processing

Increasingly it is possible to export the results of searches carried out on the clinical system to a DOS file for further processing and reporting. The most useful outcome of this is that data can be imported in a spreadsheet such as Excel, from where it can be converted into charts and graphs. This is particularly useful, as currently the output option of clinical systems, in terms of graphics, is fairly limited

Closing Summary

This chapter has been aimed at illustrating some of the issues encountered after the most basic operations of using the clinical system have been mastered. In many cases it has been necessary to concentrate on the generic, and it is very true that different systems generate different problems. If practices plan data entry carefully and are clear as to why it is taking place, and also test reporting facilities at an early stage, then things should go well.

Features specific to particular systems will be mentioned later in the chapters dedicated to specific systems.

5
The AAH Meditel System

Opening Summary

This chapter discusses the AAH Meditel System 5 computer system. It attempts to describe some of the main features of the system so that those readers who have not seen it will have a basic understanding of it. Wherever possible, screenshots have been used to show what the system looks like. It is not, and does not attempt to be, a comprehensive index of features and facilities of this system.

Basic Information

AAH Meditel System 5 is one of the most popular general practice systems currently in use, although over the next few years the majority of AAH Meditel sites are likely to change to the new AAH Meditel system, System 6000. The actual number of sites at the time of going to press is about 2000, making it the third most popular system in use.

Until recently AAH Meditel used the XENIX operating system, but has now changed over to the UNIX operating system. The system configuration is multi-user, using a central computer and a number of attached terminals. Normally these terminals are connected via one or more Specialix multiplexers. It is possible for PCs to replace terminals on the system, and in these cases terminal emulation software is used on the machine. This allows the PC to behave (while attached to the AAH Meditel system) very much like a terminal, with the exception that if the PC has a colour monitor, then certain parts of the AAH Meditel system are displayed in colour. The use of UNIX with AAH Meditel now means that this system can also be set up to work on a local area network (LAN).

Hardware is normally supplied through AAH Meditel, originating from either Dell or Compaq. Extras available include the development version of SOPHIE – the template/protocol generator, fundholding software and terminal emulation software. AAH Meditel has developed registration and IOS links software, and this is in use at a large number of practices. General practice provider links, such as pathology, are also available.

The typing in of a letter (or letters) accesses items on the main menu.

In some cases further menus will appear with different letter codes to access functions. If users know the letter code to operate a particular function then they can often access it directly without going via the menu system.

After logging into the system, the main menu is displayed, as shown in Figure 5 for a typical system.

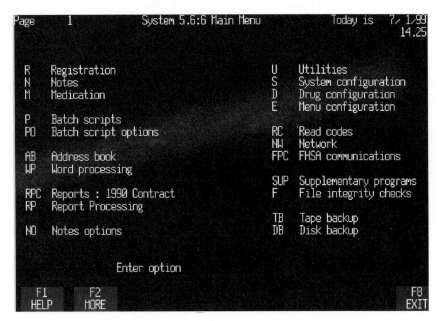

Figure 5 The AAH Meditel main menu screen

Registration

After pressing the R key, the user is presented with the registration screen show in the Figure 6. An action is then selected using the function keys. For example, new patients are added using the F4 key. When this is done, the main screen stays the same, but the action of some of the function keys changes. This is the case throughout AAH Meditel, with some function keys changing action depending on context. As with most current systems, the addition of family groups sharing a common address is made very easy. As AAH Meditel is a number-based system, it is important that the computer number is written in a prominent position on the notes. Normally the number that AAH Meditel generates should be accepted. If a different number is required, it can be entered, but it must be unique.

The AAH Meditel System   69

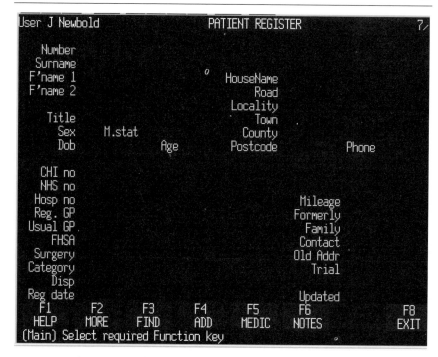

Figure 6 The AAH Meditel registration screen

To register a patient, the various fields are completed In some cases data items are compulsory, i.e. surname. Also, within certain fields pressing a function key will present the user with a picklist to choose from, i.e. for items such as GPs in the practice, and surgeries. Addresses can also be entered quickly using the address dictionary feature. The screen can be navigated using the cursor keys.

Generally the entry of data on to this screen is straightforward and it is possible to use this screen during the consultation. Note that in the initial screen, function keys allow the user to move directly to the Notes or Medication screens. Users who register a lot of patients using AAH Meditel find that the screen is very workable in practice.

Notes

The notes screen is accessed by pressing N from the main menu (it can also be accessed from other parts of the program, such as registration) and such is the importance of this area to GPs that we will look at how it operates in some detail.

On entering the notes and medication program the screen shown in Figure 7 is displayed.

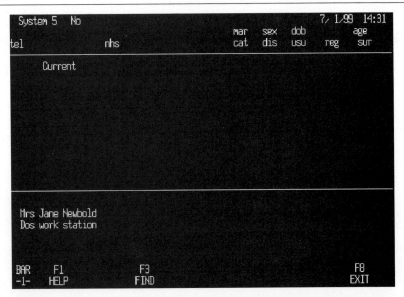

Figure 7 The AAH Meditel notes and medication screen – no patient selected

To find a patient, the function key F3 is pressed and then the AAH Meditel number can be entered, if available. If it is not available then the down arrow key can be pressed and the surname and/or initials can be entered and the patient selected from a list.

Having selected a patient, the clinical history can be reviewed using several views provided by AAH Meditel. The screen with a patient selected is shown in Figure 8.

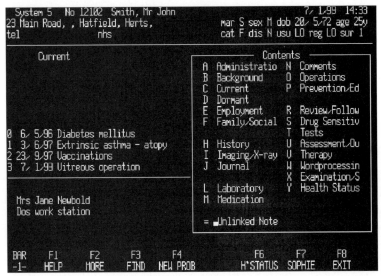

Figure 8 The AAH Meditel notes screen with a patient selected

The AAH Meditel System 71

The current section is active and shows a list of current problem titles. The AAH Meditel system divides entries into various categories or note types as shown in the contents box (all entries can be shown using the Journal option). Those options that are highlighted indicate the presence of data. Problems that are of current importance are placed in the current screen – hence its name. Note that there is an equivalent section called Dormant for non-current entries.

Entries added to the medical record consist of a Read-coded item, with optionally free text to qualify it further, together with some other details, such as the episode type, place of procedure and, in most cases, a recall date. Some Read codes, where appropriate, will prompt for a numeric value as well.

Prescribing can be actioned directly from the notes area of the program. Free text added can only be searched in a rather limited way, and is most useful for qualifying the Read-coded entries. These entries are made by typing in the first few letters of the desired term and then picking the appropriate item from a list. If the code chosen has lower level codes, then further picking lists of subcodes appear. It is possible with this system to enter Read codes directly, provided they are prefixed by a dot.

AAH Meditel uses a problem-oriented approach to the clinical record with entries normally being made under problem headings.

Problems and Problem Headings

A problem heading in AAH Meditel is rather like a container into which note entries can be placed. Another way of thinking of it is as a summary item. In order to explain it fully, we will take the example of extrinsic asthma. This can be seen in Figure 8.

The first time the patient came to see the GP a new problem was started. The new problem title was a Read code selected by entering part of a name of the condition (*extrinsic asthma*) and could be either a morbidity (if known) or a symptom. In this particular case the diagnosis was extrinsic asthma, which has the Read code H431. (This is a subcode of asthma – Read code H43.) It is possible to qualify the Read code used with free text, but in the case of a problem heading, this should normally be avoided to improve readability.

Figure 9 shows this problem exploded so that all the items relating to it can be seen. This screen shows a peak flow entry highlighted.

Note the fact that the note type of the entry is 'T'. This means 'test' and is the *type* associated with this Read code. Each Read code has a type, and an alternative way of looking at the entered data is under its particular note type. The types are shown on the previous figure under Contents (Figure 8). Pressing the letter denoting the type from the opening screen accesses each category or type. Under Tests, for example, all the Read-coded entries which were tests would appear as a list irrespective of the problem heading to which they relate. Although it is also possible to enter data while in a particular category, e.g. Tests, the entry is then not related to its particular problem. This means that if the entry of a peak flow is made under the test category, then when the problem 'Extrinsic Asthma' is viewed, this test result will not appear as one of the entries for this problem. Entering the data under the appropriate problem heading means that the data is available both as part of the problem and as an entry under the appropriate category.

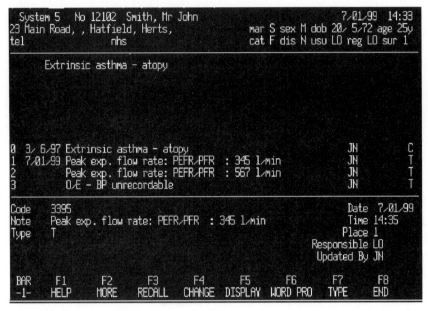

Figure 9 The AAH Meditel notes screen – medication

As well as morbidity and test data, most other entries can be made in the same way. Medication issued as a response to a particular problem can be entered within the problem and will still appear if the Medication Type screen is selected. The converse is clearly not true, and medication entered directly on to the medication screen will not be linked to any particular problem.

A significant number of AAH Meditel practices do not use the notes screen correctly, and instead enter each new *occurrence* of the problem as a new problem. The problem with this approach is that it is then difficult to look at a particular problem in isolation, as all the clinical note entries form a long list that is not structured.

Medication

AAH Meditel uses the Multilex Read-coded drug dictionary, and drugs, like other Read items, can be accessed by typing in part of their name and then picking from a list. In the case of drugs, if a code is to be typed in it must be prefixed by a comma.

Figure 10 shows a medication entry being added to AAH Meditel. Once the drug has been selected it is very simple to select the other details. The normal dose is entered for the user, but can be overwritten. Advice can also be entered. Acute and repeat medication is differentiated by an 'A' or an 'R' in the field labelled Type. If the item is a repeat then the number of scripts authorised must be filled in. Sensitivities, contraindications and interactions are supported. The issuing of prescriptions is simply a matter of marking the desired items and then pressing a function key. Generic substitution is supported via a function key.

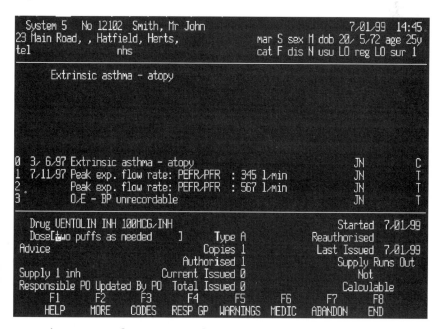

Figure 10   The AAH Meditel notes screen – medication

SOPHIE

SOPHIE is AAH Meditel's templating/protocol system and allows the user to use screens dedicated to a particular topic of data entry. The reasons for using templates were discussed previously. SOPHIE is supplied in a 'run-time' form with the standard system and users have the option to buy the 'Developers' version. This allows them to develop their own templates rather than just using those supplied by AAH Meditel. SOPHIE templates are quite powerful compared to those supplied by some other manufacturers, but are relatively complicated to produce – although very easy to use. Prompts can be age dependent or sex dependent and the need to add missing data can be highlighted. In those practices that do have the Developers version of SOPHIE it is common to find only one or two individuals able to use it – or even none at all! Users without the Developers version can obtain templates from a variety of sources, such as the user group.

Templates are most commonly used for things such as asthma, diabetes and health promotion information, and provide a way of achieving consistent and convenient data entry for relatively large amounts of information. In the example given in Figure 11 the diabetic template has been started and the user is being asked to pick an option: SOPHIE, unlike some competing systems, allows information to be extracted from existing medical records in a precise way. This information is not limited to medical history, but includes drugs, etc.

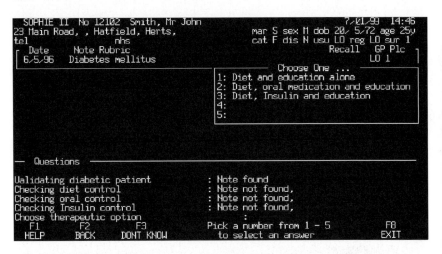

Figure 11   The AAH Meditel template/protocol screen (SOPHIE)

To enter all the same information contained in the template directly into the notes screen would normally take much longer, as each item of information would have to be entered separately. As well as this there is a good chance that at some stage a different Read code might be used to record one of the items, leading to difficulties when the information is searched.

The author has visited a number of practices that have been

entering all of their basic health information as individual entries into the notes screen. If entered with care, this will produce the desired result, but the time-saving achieved by using a SOPHIE screen is very significant.

Reporting

Reporting in AAH Meditel falls into two categories:

- Standard reports
- User-defined reports.

Standard reports are available in most areas and are extremely easy to use. Generally it is a question of selecting the desired report and supplying the required parameters to run it, i.e. the date range. Examples of standard reports provided by AAH Meditel are those on cytology targets and immunisations.

As an illustration, the options available for cytology and immunisation reports are shown in Figure 12. Figure 13 shows the cytology options available.

```
Page    22                    1990 Contract Reports      Today is    7/01/99
                                                                     14.48

        Screening and Prevention                  Activity Analysis
   RA5  Surveillance - Childhood            RC5  Prescribing Data
   RA6  Surveillance - Adult                RC6  Morbidity Data
   RA7  Surveillance - Geriatric            RC8  Referral Data
                                            RC9  Investigation Data
   RB1  Health Promotion Clinics
                                                 Registration Information
   RB3  Cervical Smear Cytology
   RB4  Immunisations - Primary             RD4  Capitation Statistics
   RB5  Immunisations - Pre-School          RD5  New Registrations
   RB6  Immunisations - Adult               RD6  Registration Categories
   RB7  Items of Service Claims             RD7  Rural Mileage
    21  Previous Menu                        23  Next Menu

                        Enter option  ■

    F1          F2          F3                                          F8
   HELP        MORE       PAGE 1                                       EXIT
```

Figure 12   The AAH Meditel cytology and immunisations reports available

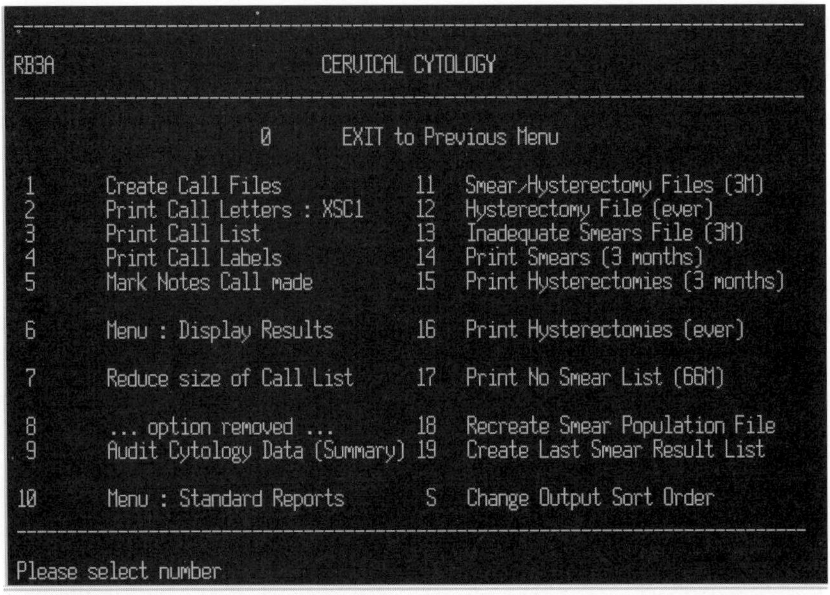

```
RB3A                    CERVICAL CYTOLOGY

                0       EXIT to Previous Menu

        1   Create Call Files            11  Smear/Hysterectomy Files (3M)
        2   Print Call Letters : XSC1    12  Hysterectomy File (ever)
        3   Print Call List              13  Inadequate Smears File (3M)
        4   Print Call Labels            14  Print Smears (3 months)
        5   Mark Notes Call made         15  Print Hysterectomies (3 months)

        6   Menu : Display Results       16  Print Hysterectomies (ever)

        7   Reduce size of Call List     17  Print No Smear List (66M)

        8       ... option removed ...   18  Recreate Smear Population File
        9   Audit Cytology Data (Summary) 19 Create Last Smear Result List

        10  Menu : Standard Reports       S  Change Output Sort Order

Please select number
```

Figure 13   The AAH Meditel cytology reporting options

The Report Generators

The report generators in AAH Meditel allow the user to construct complex queries and output the results in a variety of formats. Output from one of them can often be used as input to another, making for a powerful, if complex, system. The report generators are:

- RR – the main (and original) report generator for Read-coded data.
- ANA – the system for reporting on numerical data.
- FAR – flexible analysis reports which can provide information on the number of times a particular Read code has been used between two dates (normally used for referral analysis. All these systems are powerful, but we will concentrate on describing the use of RR, which is still the most popular way of extracting data from AAH Meditel. The RR screen is shown in Figure 14.

The screen is divided into three parts: input, processing and output. The first field on the input section is the From index.

From Index...

AAH Meditel allows searches to be carried out on a number of indexes (see Chapter 4). There are several index types that can be searched including Read codes, encounter dates and recall dates. In order to search using a particular index, in most cases a *selection group* has to be set up. The exception to this rule is in the case of the 'Medical Read code *Quick*', which allows searches to be carried out simply by using a particular Read code as the criterion.

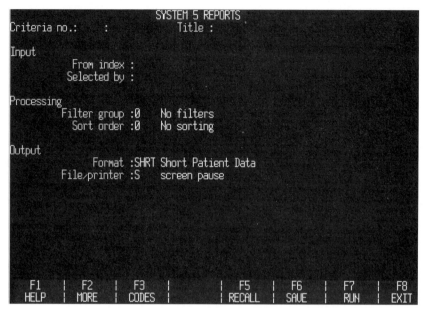

Figure 14 The AAH Meditel report generator

A search for people with asthma recorded in the last two years could be carried out by setting up a selection group using the encounter date index which selects records on the basis of the Read codes recorded and the date of the encounter. The setting up of the selection group is done either by using the selection code editor or by using a previously stored selection group for that index. This may seem complicated at first, but once the process has been used a few times, it becomes a lot easier. Figure 15 shows the editor being used to set up a selection criteria.

Many searches can be run on the basis of indexes alone, but in some cases it may be necessary to select patients further on the basis of other criteria as well. In this case filters are very useful.

Filters

Filters are a secondary method of selecting records during a search. They take the records selected by an index according to the selection criteria and subject them to further criteria according to the *filter group* in use. Filters are much slower in operation than indexes because they evaluate every record that is passed to them. Having said this, it is the combination of indexed and filtered searches that gives AAH Meditel its great flexibility in selecting patient records.

```
System 5              Report by encounter date                 7/01/99

    Report range code :AJR1:     title :BPs last 3 years


    Encounter date during Last  3  Years  Last This) no. (D W M Q Y)
    With Read codes in one of the ranges below
    from: 2466: O/E - BP reading raised      to: 2467: O/E - BP reading very high
        :       :                                :        :
        :       :                                :        :
    ┌─────────────────────────────────────────────────────┐
    │ 0  AELL   A & E LM                                  │
    │ 1  AJR1   BPs last 3 years                          │
    │ 2  CE3!   Child Examination L 3 Months              │
    │ 3  CFQ!   Claim Form Last 3 Months                  │
    │ 4  CFY!   Claim Form Last 12 Months                 │
    │ 5  CHLL   chiropody clinic                          │
    │ 6  CL3!   Child Call 9061 Last 6 Weeks              │
    │ 7  CNH!   H/O Cx neoplasia L120M                    │
    │ 8  CON    contraception                             │
    │ 9  CRE!   Child Surv. Reg. Status L3M               │
    └─────────────────────────────────────────────────────┘
    │  F1   │  F2   │  F3   │  F4   │  F5    │       │  F7    │  F8   │
    │ HELP  │ MORE  │ FIND  │ ADD   │ CHANGE │       │ DELETE │ EXIT  │
```

Figure 15   The AAH Meditel selection criteria for report

Filters are individual criteria that are used to select records. They can be based on criteria selected from any of the main areas of the AAH Meditel system. Before filters can be used, they are combined together into filter groups. By maintaining a number of different filters (which can be created by a process similar to creating selection groups mentioned earlier), a much larger number of filter groups can be made by effectively adding and subtracting the effect of the individual filters. In practice, many filtered searches consist of filter groups which contain just one filter.

It can be imagined that coming to grips with these concepts takes a certain amount of application, but having done so, very complex searches can then be devised.

Sort Order, Format and Output

Having selected the required patient records, using either an index or a combination of an index and a filter, the selected records can be sorted into any of a number of orders. For example, they could be put in surname order. Apart from the convenience of having the records in a particular order, the use of a sort order ensures that records will not be counted twice. This can happen if no sort order is used and the particular criteria being searched appears twice in a patient's notes.

A wide range of output formats can be used for the selected patients. One of the simplest would be a straight count. Another would be the patients' names and addresses. Many other output options are possible including sophisticated ones that will pull out data from the records of the selected patients and those that will produce histograms or age-banded output.

The final option on the main (RR) screen allows the report to be directed to a variety of output devices including the screen, printers and files. In cases where AAH Meditel is being used on a PC it is here that the option exists to send the report to a DOS format ASCII file.

Recent Changes

Recently a number of new features have been added to the AAH Meditel system, including such things as patient advice leaflets (PALs). A new appointment system is also to be released soon. There are a number of third-party programs available for use with AAH Meditel System 5. The most popular of these is the 'Frontdesk' appointment system from Doctors Independent Network. This fully featured appointment system is fully integrated with System 5 and is very popular with GPs and staff. In parallel with System 5, an entirely new Windows-based system has been developed that will be discussed briefly in Chapter 8. It is likely that significant numbers of AAH Meditel users will migrate to the new system at some point in the future.

Closing Summary

> AAH Meditel is a comprehensive medical system that will fulfil all the main requirements of a general practice. Its main strengths are its very flexible medical record – particularly the strong problem orientation with the ability to look at the information in a variety of ways – and its powerful report generator. At first sight the reporting can be a little complicated, particularly if a complex report has to be produced. In addition, setting up SOPHIE protocols can be complex (although it is very easy to use). AAH Meditel is still one of the leading systems currently available.

At a glance: The AAH Meditel *System 5*

Strengths	Features	Ratings (on a scale of 1–10)
A well respected system from a major supplier that is capable of most tasks. Powerful reporting and a very strongly problem-oriented record make this system a good contender for those practices wishing to store full clinical details of consultations, etc.	Administration/ registration data	✔✔✔✔✔✔✔
	Consultation data	✔✔✔✔✔✔✔
	Reporting	✔✔✔✔✔✔✔✔
	Templates	✔✔✔✔✔✔
	Integration	✔✔✔✔✔✔✔
	Look and feel	✔✔✔✔✔
	Costs	✔✔✔
	Support	✔✔✔✔✔✔
	Overall	✔✔✔✔✔✔✔✔✔

Weaknesses

Old fashioned compared with the new System 6000.

Can be difficult to get to grips with at first.

6
The EMIS System

Opening Summary

This chapter discusses the EMIS clinical computer system. It attempts to describe some of the main features of the system so that those readers who have not seen it will at least have a basic impression of it. Wherever possible screenshots have been used to show what the system looks like. It is not, and does not attempt to be, a comprehensive index of features and facilities of this system.

Basic Information

EMIS has been a very successful company in the last few years and its user base has expanded such that it is now, with VAMP and AAH Meditel, one of the 'big three' suppliers, with approximately 2500 sites. EMIS are in the process of developing a new 'GUI' version of the system, but few details of this had been released at the time of writing. Although not having as many sites as VAMP, EMIS is the largest single system on the market (VAMP sites are a mixture of VAMP Medical, VAMP Vision, Surgery Manager and GP Plus).

EMIS uses the MUMPS operating system, which runs 'on top of' MS-DOS, and the system configuration is multi-user, using a central computer and a number of attached terminals that are normally connected via one or more Arnet multiplexers. PCs can replace terminals on the system, in which case terminal-emulation software is used on the it, and it behaves (while attached to the EMIS system) very much like a terminal. The only difference is that if the PC has a colour monitor, then certain parts of the EMIS system are displayed in colour. Recent EMIS installations have been of the network type, using a version of MUMPS running with Windows NT Server.

Hardware is normally supplied by EMIS and was formerly of their own brand name. It is now normally either Hewlett Packard or another established supplier. Available extras are few, as the EMIS system already includes the template generator, and an accounting package. An expert system called MENTOR is also included and EMIS have involved many practices in the Prodigy prescribing project. They have developed GP–HA links software and this is in use at a large number of practices. IOS and pathology links software are also available and widely used.

A fairly basic word processing package is included that can directly import aspects of the patient record to ease writing referral letters. There are also a number of patient information leaflets (PILs) that can be printed by the word processor.

The current EMIS system is text based and the new Windows-based front end is expected ultimately to replace the present system. In the interim a new series of terminal emulator programs have been launched to make the program easier to use from a Windows environment.

Items on the main menu are accessed in a similar way to AAH Meditel, i.e. by typing in letters such as CM for consultation mode, etc. As well as this, considerable use is made of the function keys, which have a consistent meaning throughout the program. After logging on to the system, the opening menu is displayed. This is shown in Figure 16.

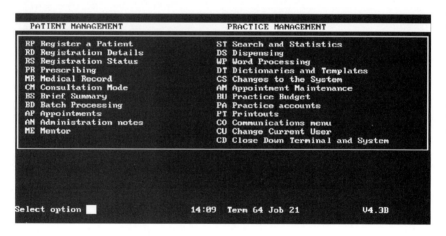

Figure 16   The EMIS main menu

Registration

Registration in EMIS is very straightforward. On selecting the appropriate option (RP) you are prompted to choose the registration type, e.g. regular, temporary, etc and then the main registration screen is shown (Figure 17).

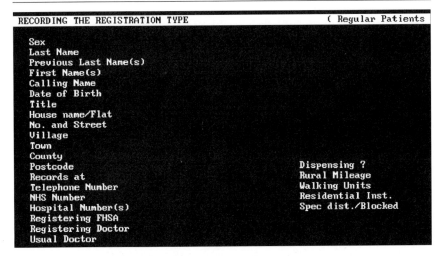

Figure 17   The EMIS registration screen

Data is entered using the 'Find' key (F4) to access the list of addresses already on file. If a date of birth is entered which is already on file you are asked if you are entering a duplicate record. This allows the easy checking of patients who have left and are now re-registering. If you are entering many members of the same family you can choose to default to the previous address entered. The 'Find' key that accesses the internal dictionaries is not mandatory, which makes for speed of data entry at the expense of data accuracy. As EMIS uses a number unique to each patient, it is useful to write this number on the notes for reference.

Medical Record

The medical record in EMIS is extremely flexible. Broadly there are three methods of entering data for an individual patient, although the methods overlap. Loosely these are:

- Medical record (MR).
- Templates (and protocols).
- Consultation mode (CM).

Medical Record Mode

Patients can be selected at any point in the system by record number, name, address, date of birth or telephone number, etc. EMIS is unique in that it assesses the type of data that you have entered, rather than requiring different fields to be entered. In practice this means very rapid selection of patients. If there is a match, you will be asked if this is the correct patient. Otherwise you will be given a picking list or be told that there is no match. Figure 18 shows the main screen in MR mode.

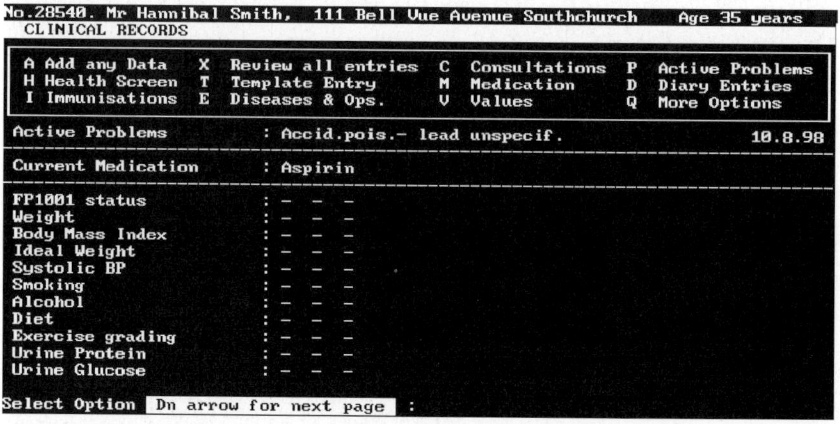

```
No.28540. Mr Hannibal Smith,   111 Bell Vue Avenue Southchurch    Age 35 years
   CLINICAL RECORDS
┌─────────────────────────────────────────────────────────────────────────────┐
│ A  Add any Data      X  Review all entries   C  Consultations   P  Active Problems │
│ H  Health Screen     T  Template Entry       M  Medication      D  Diary Entries   │
│ I  Immunisations     E  Diseases & Ops.      V  Values          Q  More Options    │
├─────────────────────────────────────────────────────────────────────────────┤
│ Active Problems          : Accid.pois.- lead unspecif.               10.8.98 │
│ Current Medication       : Aspirin                                           │
├─────────────────────────────────────────────────────────────────────────────┤
│ FP1001 status            : - - -                                             │
│ Weight                   : - - -                                             │
│ Body Mass Index          : - - -                                             │
│ Ideal Weight             : - - -                                             │
│ Systolic BP              : - - -                                             │
│ Smoking                  : - - -                                             │
│ Alcohol                  : - - -                                             │
│ Diet                     : - - -                                             │
│ Exercise grading         : - - -                                             │
│ Urine Protein            : - - -                                             │
│ Urine Glucose            : - - -                                             │
├─────────────────────────────────────────────────────────────────────────────┤
│ Select Option  Dn arrow for next page  :                                     │
└─────────────────────────────────────────────────────────────────────────────┘
```

Figure 18 The EMIS medical record screen

EMIS allows you to enter data in two ways. The first is by searchable Read codes. The second is via free text that cannot be searched. It is possible to insert any number of Read codes into a block of free text, and, of course, these can subsequently be retrieved in a search. In practice this can be very convenient. The simplest screen for data entry is the 'add any data screen' (Figure 19).

This screen is useful for entering summary data. At the prompt 'Make your entry here' you can enter a Read code, a description of a Read code or a partial description or code. The items A–Y shown are shortcuts to various categories of code *and the user can amend these shortcuts*. You are invited to choose a Read code and then to add a few comments in free text. All entries will appear not only in this screen, but also in any relevant part of any other screen.

All entries can be deemed as *active* or *inactive* problems. In practical terms, an active problem is highlighted on the summary screen, whereas an inactive problem is not. It is possible to activate and de-activate problems at any time.

Consultation Mode (CM)

Consultation mode is the main way in which GPs enter data into EMIS. When entered (using the code CM) there is an option of being shown a brief summary screen before entering the patient details. After this the main consultation screen shown in Figure 20 appears.

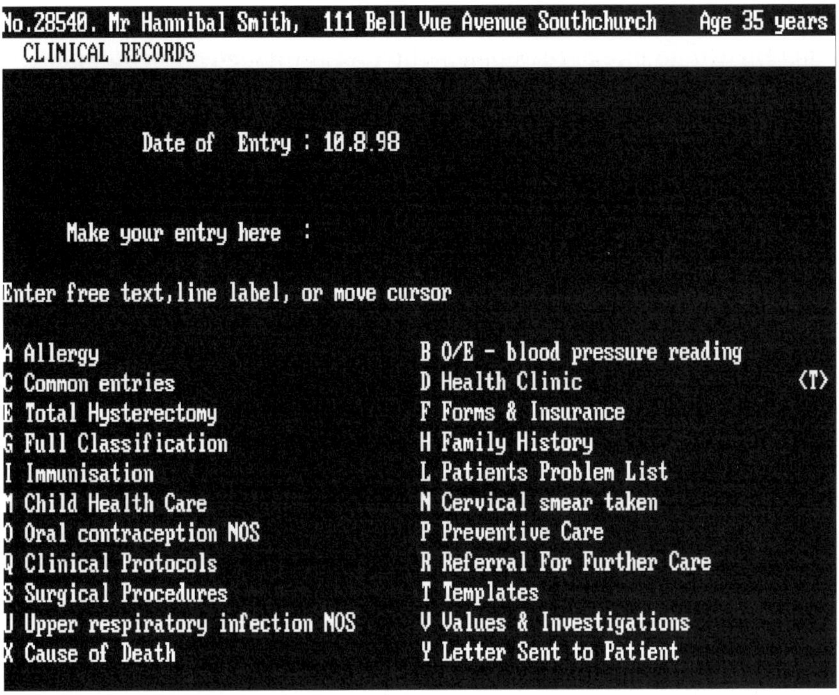

The EMIS System 85

```
No.28540. Mr Hannibal Smith,  111 Bell Vue Avenue Southchurch    Age 35 years
CLINICAL RECORDS


            Date of  Entry : 10.8.98


       Make your entry here  :

Enter free text, line label, or move cursor

A Allergy                         B O/E - blood pressure reading
C Common entries                  D Health Clinic                  (T)
E Total Hysterectomy              F Forms & Insurance
G Full Classification             H Family History
I Immunisation                    L Patients Problem List
M Child Health Care               N Cervical smear taken
O Oral contraception NOS          P Preventive Care
Q Clinical Protocols              R Referral For Further Care
S Surgical Procedures             T Templates
U Upper respiratory infection NOS V Values & Investigations
X Cause of Death                  Y Letter Sent to Patient
```

Figure 19   Adding clinical data in EMIS

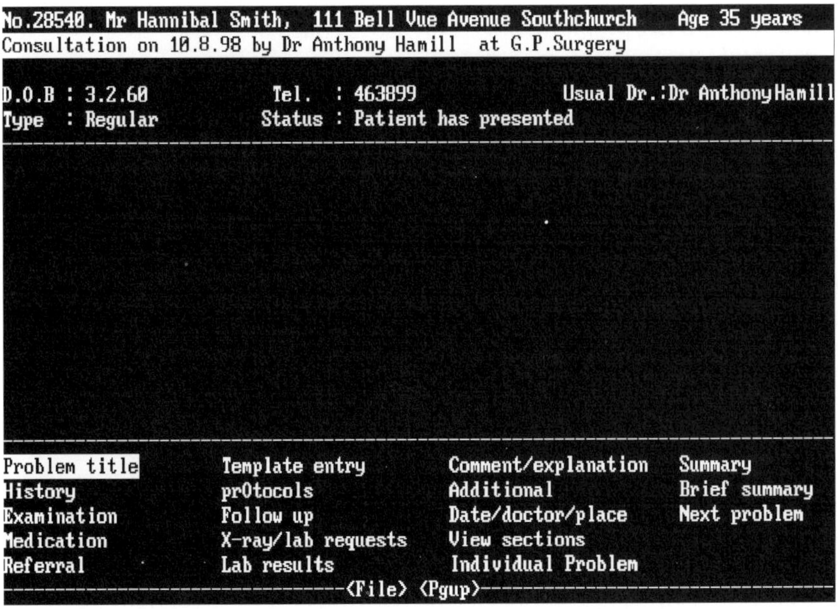

```
No.28540. Mr Hannibal Smith,  111 Bell Vue Avenue Southchurch    Age 35 years
Consultation on 10.8.98 by Dr Anthony Hamill   at G.P.Surgery

D.O.B : 3.2.60          Tel.  : 463899           Usual Dr.:Dr AnthonyHamill
Type  : Regular         Status : Patient has presented









Problem title      Template entry       Comment/explanation   Summary
History            pr0tocols            Additional            Brief summary
Examination        Follow up            Date/doctor/place     Next problem
Medication         X-ray/lab requests   View sections
Referral           Lab results          Individual Problem
------------------------------<File> <Pgup>-------------------------------
```

Figure 20   The consultation mode screen

The menu at the bottom of the screen shows the options. After entering data in one of the options the user is prompted to enter data in the next option. It is possible to alter the sequence in which these options occur. Values (measured or biochemical) are entered under the View Sections / Values screen (see later) or directly using the 'Find' key. If the surgery is using Lablinks this is where the electronically entered data can be viewed.

'Problems' in EMIS

Problems in EMIS are handled in a rather different way from those in AAH Meditel. They are defined by using the Problem Title option shown in Figure 20. This leads to the screen shown in Figure 19, from which a Read code can be selected.

Once a problem has been defined for a patient, further entries for the same problem can be made by either:

- Selecting the same problem title
  or
- Selecting the problem from the patients problem list, which inserts the same problem title (this list is accessible from the screen shown in Figure 19).

In this way problems are made up from consultation entries which share a common problem title. This is in contrast to the AAH Meditel system in which, once a problem has been defined, other entries are made under this heading.

Before leaving the topic of problem titles it should be mentioned that EMIS does not force the use of a Read code as a problem title. It is possible to enter free text instead, but then this data cannot be searched and the item cannot be properly structured.

Once the problem title has been entered, history and examination data (free text) can be entered. From within the free text sections it is possible to enter a Read code by pressing the versatile 'Find' key, which again brings up the screen shown in Figure 19. Entering data such as blood pressure is best done this way. Writing BP 125/65 in free text is only of use when viewing the particular record it is written in. To view it later with all the other readings it must be Read coded.

Medication

Medication can be prescribed directly from the CM screen, and in general this is usually the most convenient way of doing it, with the added advantage of being able to keep a record of it together with other details of the consultation. Alternatively, medication can be accessed directly from the main menu without going via the CM screen, although this means that it is not directly related to the condition for which it is prescribed. This functionality is similar to AAH Meditel, where the same two methods of setting up prescriptions exist (see Chapter 5).

Figure 21 shows aspirin being selected for prescription. All the normal features are present including contraindications and easy swapping to generic forms. Of note is the feature which will automatically promote the most commonly used form of a drug to the top of the picking list and a useful feature that allows very quick selection of the dose information (based on previous use) once a drug has been selected. Figure 22 shows a partially completed consultation screen after the medication has been added.

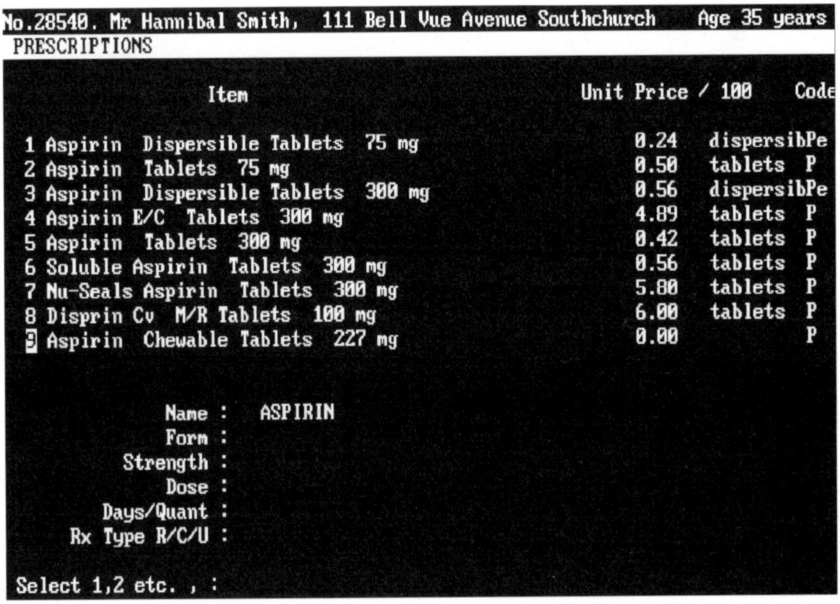

```
No.28540. Mr Hannibal Smith,  111 Bell Vue Avenue Southchurch    Age 35 years
PRESCRIPTIONS

                Item                        Unit Price / 100    Code

1 Aspirin  Dispersible Tablets   75 mg           0.24      dispersibPe
2 Aspirin  Tablets   75 mg                       0.50      tablets   P
3 Aspirin  Dispersible Tablets  300 mg           0.56      dispersibPe
4 Aspirin  E/C Tablets  300 mg                   4.89      tablets   P
5 Aspirin  Tablets  300 mg                       0.42      tablets   P
6 Soluble Aspirin  Tablets  300 mg               0.56      tablets   P
7 Nu-Seals Aspirin  Tablets  300 mg              5.00      tablets   P
8 Disprin Cv M/R Tablets  100 mg                 6.00      tablets   P
9 Aspirin  Chewable Tablets  227 mg              0.00                P


            Name :   ASPIRIN
            Form :
        Strength :
            Dose :
      Days/Quant :
     Rx Type R/C/U :

Select 1,2 etc. , :
```

Figure 21   The EMIS prescribing screen

There are many other options on this screen. From within consultation mode it is possible to log referrals to other agencies, put in diary entries for follow-ups and monitor laboratory requests and results. If the data is Read coded it can be searched later.

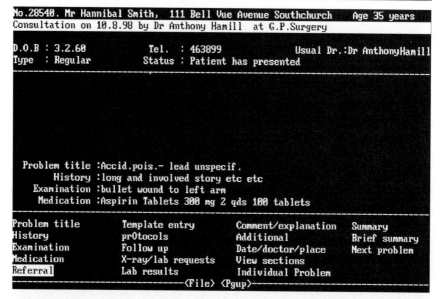

Figure 22 A consultation showing the medication prescribed

Overall, the CM screen is very powerful and can be used as little or as much as a particular practice decides. Most GPs find that once they are familiar with this screen they can carry out 95% of all data entry from it. The problem-oriented features are not as strong as with AAH Meditel but it is better in terms of its ability to record a number of Read-coded items both logically and easily.

Templates

Another highly structured method of entering data is via templates (and protocols). Templates are similar to SOPHIE screens in AAH Meditel. Within EMIS the templating system is highly integrated, with templates being available from both the main data entry screens (Medical Record and Consultation Mode). A simple template is shown below. This is the supplied Health Screen template that is accessed from the MR menu (Figure 23).

Templates in EMIS are data entry forms. They do not branch, as is the case with SOPHIE (protocols do this in EMIS). They are, however, extremely easy to set up and it is quite easy for a practice to modify or create a completely new template for a particular purpose. Templates in EMIS can only have Read codes as the basis of the fields in the form. At first sight this can be seen as a disadvantage, but fits in with the ability of EMIS to search on Read-coded data only. Depending on how a template is built, it can be automatically triggered by selecting a Read code when entering data. For example, if asthma is entered as a new problem title, this will prompt the system to ask if the appropriate template should be run.

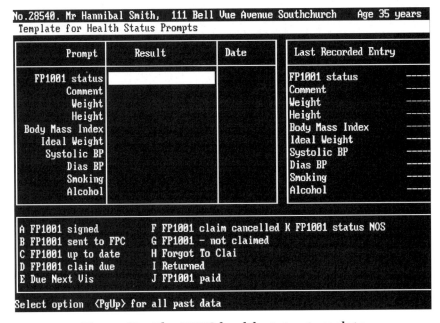

Figure 23 The EMIS health status template

Protocols are in some ways similar to templates in that they collect data, but protocols are a far more powerful tool, supporting branching (like SOPHIE in AAH Meditel), while sharing many of the same features. They are also much more difficult to set up, although the results can be very worthwhile. They can also be attached to a Read code in the same way as templates.

Reporting

Reporting in EMIS is powerful and relatively straightforward, even for the beginner. It differs substantially from searching in AAH Meditel both in philosophy and practice, in that there is no separate searching facility for numeric information – all information Read codes and numerics are accessed via one screen. Additionally, the topic of indexing is irrelevant to the user as methods of searching are all handled internally. Apart from the usual standard reports there are essentially two main types of report in EMIS:

- Patient searches
- Audit searches

Patient Searches

On selecting patient searches, a screen containing options to build new searches, look at search results, edit searches, etc is displayed (Figure 24). If a new search is selected, the user selects features for the search by adding them to the screen (Figure 25). It is fairly easy to build up complex searches involving many parameters, although clearly the speed of searching drops off as searches become more complex. Boolean (AND, OR and NOT) algebra is catered for and each feature can have a date range added to it. The only type of searches that are harder to accomplish (in common with most other systems) are those looking for individuals with the greatest occurrence of a certain Read code.

In the example shown in Figure 25, a feature called 'asthma' has been added and so the search is describing currently registered patients who have a Read code for asthma in their notes. EMIS allows searching for particular Read codes or for all codes at and below a particular level.

Further features could be added to the above search until the desired result was obtained. Features, essentially elements in the search, can be combined logically. In this way, patients who have asthma and had not had a peak flow in the last year, could be found.

Having created a search there are a wide number of ways within EMIS to look at the results. Perhaps one of the best to use for a quick summery of the data is the Table option. This shows the number of males and females who were qualified by the search parameters both as numbers and as a percentage of the relevant practice population. The output, which is normally first directed to the screen, is also broken down by age band.

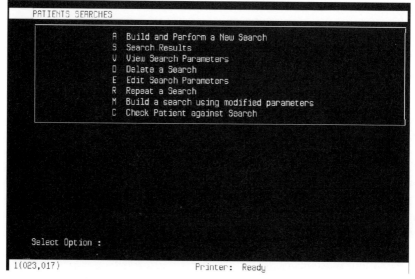

Figure 24   The main patient search menu

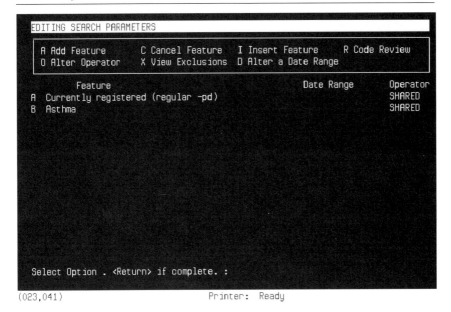

Figure 25 EMIS building a search

Other useful result options are a list of names and addresses, output showing selected parts of the medical record and output to an ASCII file (see Chapter 9). It is also easy to create a file from which the records of the patients involved can be inspected.

Audit Searches

Audit searches are more complex than ordinary searches but can produce very useful summary information on a group of patients. They carry out many related searches on a group of patients called a *target* group.

Firstly, the target group is defined. This involves a normal search to identify the patients who are in the group. Secondly, the audit search is defined by adding to it factors about this group of patients. As a simple example, an asthma audit search would be based on all those patients in the practice recorded as having the appropriate Read code for asthma (normally H33). Lines in the audit would then count how many of these patients had a peak flow in the last six months, how many had been seen in the practice, how many had been given advice, etc. These counts can be further analysed by factors such as patient age or registered GP.

The final output from an audit resembles a spreadsheet and can contain all the numerical analysis involved in carrying out successful audit.

At an advanced level this can be taken further with results based on the combination of two factors being reported.

Recent Developments

Recently EMIS has been using PCs instead of terminals as the normal choice of screen. They have developed a terminal emulation program called LV1 which allows EMIS to be run from Windows 95/98. This brings with it a number of advantages, including cut and paste, and macros.

Closing Summary

EMIS has many very useful features and can, as can AAH Meditel, be described as a comprehensive general practice system that should fulfil all the requirements of a practice. Its strengths are the flexibility and power of its medical-record and consultation-mode screens, together with its templating system (the prompts of which can be made age- and sex-sensitive). A variety of small but useful features make it very user friendly. In addition to the main features mentioned in this chapter, EMIS has a powerful integrated appointments system, internal messaging (like AAH Meditel), dispensing/stock control and fully automatic updating of the software/drug dictionary, etc via modem. Additionally, a feature called portable *EMIS allows patient records to be temporarily downloaded to a portable computer for updating on home visits, etc.*

Ultimately less rigorously problem-oriented than AAH Meditel, but with similar comprehensive searching capabilities, it cannot be said to be either superior or inferior to it – merely different. Like AAH Meditel, those GPs who wish to enter large amounts of clinical data favour it. It is currently the system with the largest number of paperless practices.

In contrast to the other two 'big' suppliers, EMIS has not yet announced final details of its new graphically based system, but it is to be hoped that as much attention is paid to the detailed usability as in the present system.

The EMIS System

At a glance: **EMIS**

Strengths	Features	Ratings (on a scale of 1–10)
Another leading system – EMIS's strengths are the very consistent feel of the program throughout, coupled with the ease of use and very powerful features. A favourite with paperless practices.	Administration/ registration data Consultation data Reporting Templates Integration Look and feel Costs Support Overall	✓✓✓✓✓✓✓ ✓✓✓✓✓✓✓✓ ✓✓✓✓✓✓✓✓ ✓✓✓✓✓✓✓✓ ✓✓✓✓✓✓✓✓ ✓✓✓✓ ✓✓✓ ✓✓✓✓✓✓ ✓✓✓✓✓✓✓

Weaknesses

It looks a little old fashioned compared to the new Windows-based programs and the problem orientation is less strong than in Meditel System 5.

7
The VAMP Medical System

Opening Summary

This chapter discusses the VAMP Medical computer system. It attempts to describe some of the main features of the system so that those readers who have not previously encountered it will have an idea of it. Wherever possible, screenshots have been used to show how the system appears. It is not, and does not attempt to be, a comprehensive index of features and facilities of this system.

Basic Information

The VAMP Medical system has been in operation for several years and is still in very widespread use. It is gradually being replaced by the new Vamp Vision system, but will be around for some years yet. Recently it has been updated, and Read codes, as opposed to OXMIS codes, are now available. (The Vamp Vision system is briefly described in a later chapter.)

The exact number of sites is unclear, but it is probably in excess of 2000, making it the second most popular system in use at this time. Vamp Medical (hereafter referred to simply as 'Vamp', for convenience) is a terminal-based system that uses one main computer linked to a multiplexer to terminals (or PCs) running terminal emulation. The operating system is BOS (note that this is a completely different operating system from DOS) and it is the use of this operating system which gives the system many of its characteristics.

Vamp could not be described as the ideal system for use in the consultation as it lacks many features of the structured patient record, but, on the other hand, it is capable of carrying out all the normal administrative functions, as well as storing some patient data. One of its main benefits is that it is extremely easy to use. With the recent additions and enhancements, it should be suitable for use in small-to-medium-sized practices for quite some time.

Vamp are already well organised with regard to links, and the Vamp system can be run in conjunction with the Vamp Communicator in order to supply registration, IOS (and even pathology) links. Vamp can also supply a complete fundholding system to integrate with the clinical system, as well as many other software packages.

The main method of navigating the VAMP system is by the use of 'transactions'. The transaction prompt is a version of the command prompt, and typing in the appropriate two-letter codes accesses different screens. This means that within the clinical system there is no main menu as such, although help on what transactions are available is always accessible by means of a few key-presses.

The help on transactions is shown in Figure 26. Normally the box in the centre of the screen would not be visible, but here the help system has been activated to show some possible transactions. As there are three pages of transactions this is sometimes inconvenient, as in order to find the two-letter code for a transaction on the third page of help it is necessary to press H to get help, and then N for next page, twice!

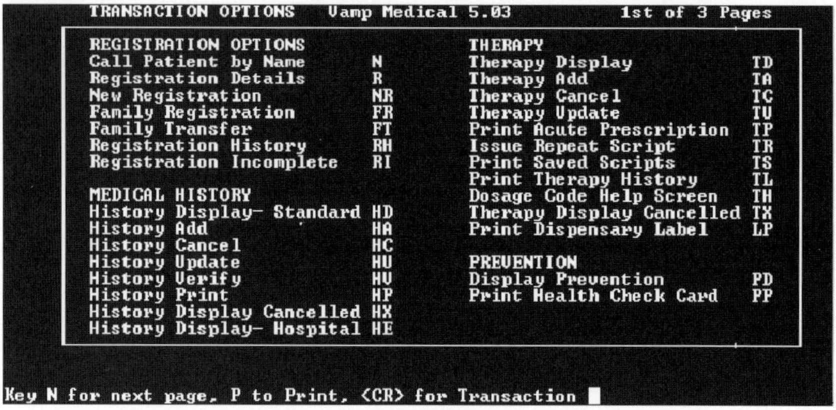

```
TRANSACTION OPTIONS    Vamp Medical 5.03           1st of 3 Pages
REGISTRATION OPTIONS                  THERAPY
Call Patient by Name      N           Therapy Display              TD
Registration Details      R           Therapy Add                  TA
New Registration          NR          Therapy Cancel               IC
Family Registration       FR          Therapy Update               TU
Family Transfer           FT          Print Acute Prescription     IP
Registration History      RH          Issue Repeat Script          IR
Registration Incomplete   RI          Print Saved Scripts          IS
                                      Print Therapy History        IL
MEDICAL HISTORY                       Dosage Code Help Screen      TH
History Display- Standard HD          Therapy Display Cancelled    TX
History Add               HA          Print Dispensary Label       LP
History Cancel            HC
History Update            HU          PREVENTION
History Verify            HV          Display Prevention           PD
History Print             HP          Print Health Check Card      PP
History Display Cancelled HX
History Display- Hospital HE

Key N for next page, P to Print, <CR> for Transaction
```

Figure 26 Examples of 'transactions' in Vamp

Registration

Vamp provides all the usual registration facilities with the opportunity to use a wide range of registration categories. The main registration screen is shown in Figure 27. Generally, registrations in Vamp are straightforward. Vamp has a strong 'family' feature which allows rapid reference to, and processing of, family units. Several of the fields have pop-up boxes showing the choices available. The screen is generally easy to use, although the choices available are not user definable. In common with other systems, some of the fields are mandatory and must be completed in order to proceed. Vamp's established registration-links facility allows for registration information to be sent and received from the HA by means of an electronic data link, and in this case the process of registration is necessarily slightly more time consuming.

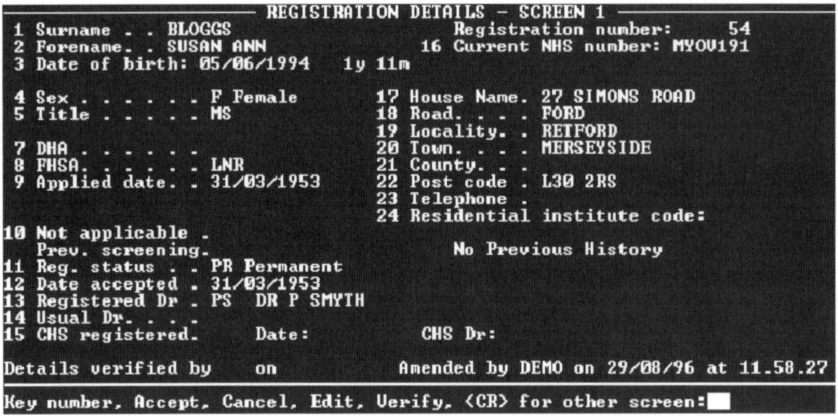

The VAMP Medical System

```
─────────────────── REGISTRATION DETAILS - SCREEN 1 ───────────────────
 1 Surname  . . BLOGGS              Registration number:      54
 2 Forename . . SUSAN ANN           16 Current NHS number: MYOU191
 3 Date of birth: 05/06/1994  1y 11m

 4 Sex . . . . . . F Female         17 House Name. 27 SIMONS ROAD
 5 Title . . . . . MS               18 Road. . . . FORD
                                    19 Locality. . RETFORD
 7 DHA . . . . . .                  20 Town. . . . MERSEYSIDE
 8 FHSA. . . . . . LNR              21 County. . .
 9 Applied date. . 31/03/1953       22 Post code . L30 2RS
                                    23 Telephone .
                                    24 Residential institute code:
10 Not applicable .
   Prev. screening.                          No Previous History
11 Reg. status . . PR Permanent
12 Date accepted . 31/03/1953
13 Registered Dr . PS  DR P SMYTH
14 Usual Dr. . . .
15 CHS registered.     Date:           CHS Dr:

Details verified by    on          Amended by DEMO on 29/08/96 at 11.58.27
Key number, Accept, Cancel, Edit, Verify, <CR> for other screen:█
```

Figure 27   The Vamp registration screen

Patient Notes

There are a variety of ways of entering patient clinical information into the Vamp system, namely:

- Prevention screen
- History screen
- Freehand

Of these, freehand is essentially a template system and as such will be dealt with under the appropriate heading.

Prevention Screen

The prevention screen is mainly of a fixed format and contains much basic patient data including items defined as major problems, height, weight, blood pressure, etc. The screen is shown in Figure 28.

In general the PD screen is well liked by both GPs and staff as it shows a summary of important basic medical information about the patient. The screen is actually a summary screen in the literal sense as 'behind' it there are all the individual records of the particular category. For example, line 5 shows the latest blood pressure reading, but by entering 5R (records), all the historical values for blood pressure can be displayed. New values can be added at either point – to the summary screen or to the screen for the particular value in question. Medical history items, which have been appropriately marked, can also be made to appear on this screen.

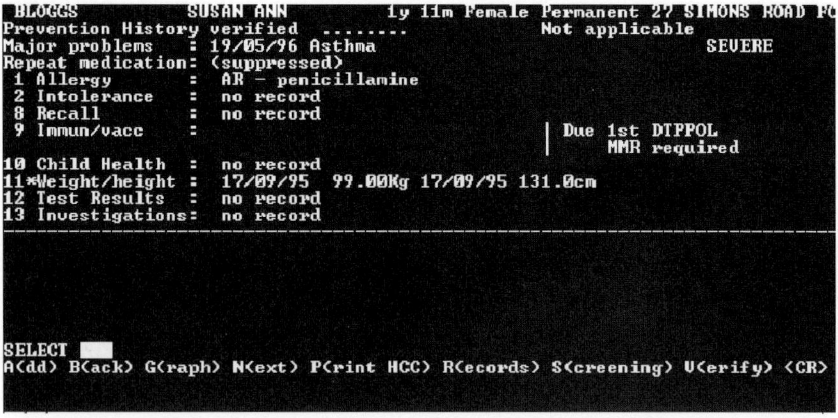

```
BLOGGS            SUSAN ANN            1y 11m Female Permanent 27 SIMONS ROAD PO
Prevention History verified   ........           Not applicable
Major problems   : 19/05/96 Asthma                                  SEVERE
Repeat medication: (suppressed)
 1 Allergy       : AR - penicillamine
 2 Intolerance   : no record
 8 Recall        : no record
 9 Immun/vacc    :                              | Due 1st DTPPOL
                                                |         MMR required
10 Child Health  : no record
11*Weight/height : 17/09/95   99.00Kg 17/09/95 131.0cm
12 Test Results  : no record
13 Investigations: no record
-------------------------------------------------------------------------



SELECT ▮
A(dd) B(ack) G(raph) N(ext) P(rint HCC) R(ecords) S(creening) U(erify) <CR>
```

Figure 28   The Vamp prevention display (PD) screen

Medical History

The medical history screen in Vamp Medical is less sophisticated than the equivalent screens in AAH Meditel and EMIS, but nevertheless is quite adequate for the basic recording of medical history data.

In order to enter data, a patient is selected using the transaction N (this is mildly confusing as N is also used to select Next Page after H Help has been selected). Patients can be selected by their surname, surname and forename or number. After selecting a patient, the user is returned to the transaction prompt. Figure 29 shows the history screen.

In simple terms an entry is first made by entering a date (or accepting the default by pressing enter). Then the type of entry is made by reference to a list – again a default can be accepted by pressing return. After this, the first part of an OXMIS term can be entered, and if the term is found, it can be accepted. If not, terms beginning with these letters can be listed. After this, the outcome can be entered (again from a list) and a free text comment (not searchable) can also be inserted. Finally, an episode type and a priority number can be entered. Of these the priority number can be useful as it can be used to filter both more important and less important items, as well as to regulate what history items appear on the PD screen. In earlier versions of Vamp, the amount of room for text comments was very limited, but this has been significantly improved in the latest version.

The VAMP Medical System

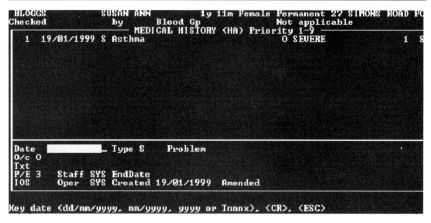

Figure 29   The Vamp history screen (later version)

Also in this latest version, Read codes can be used in preference to OXMIS and methods of ascending and descending the Read tree have been added. This change brings Vamp much more into line with other major systems.

Prescribing

Prescribing in Vamp is carried out using the various therapy options such as TA (for therapy add). Entry of a new drug is done via the Therapy Add screen, which is similar in appearance to the HA screen. The date of issue defaults to the current date (but may be altered using the Control-B key combination). After this, a part of the drug name is entered, along with (optionally) the form and strength. The drug, if found, can be selected. Similar drugs can be listed or a different form of the drug can be selected from the list. Both generic substitution and a practice-defined formulary are available as options. Once familiar with this screen, acute and repeat prescriptions are rapidly set up.

To issue a script, a different transaction (TP – therapy print) is used, and while this is also rapid in operation, initially it is a little cumbersome. There is no link with medical history, so the concept of grouping prescribing and other information together into problems is not possible. Figure 30 shows the therapy add screen.

Freehand

Freehand is the Vamp Medical template system but it is less well integrated into the rest of the system than is the case with the other two major systems. On the plus side, it is both flexible and easy to use and the reporting that can be done from freehand screens is far superior to the standard reports for the items it covers.

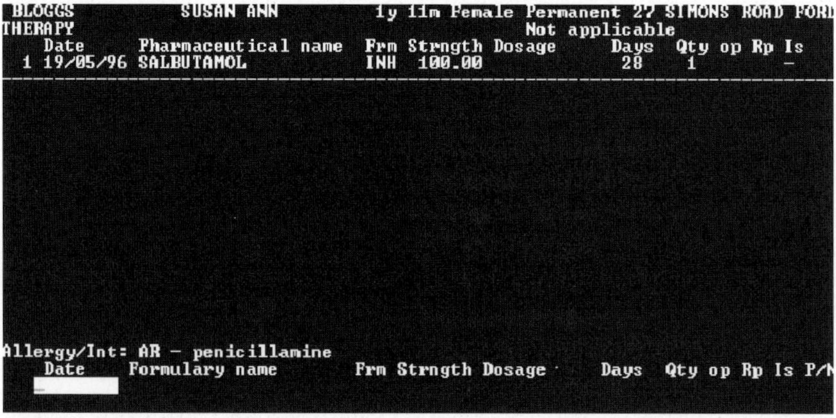

```
BLOGGS           SUSAN ANN           1y 11m Female Permanent 27 SIMONS ROAD FORD
THERAPY                                           Not applicable
    Date         Pharmaceutical name    Frm Strngth Dosage    Days    Qty op Rp Is
1 19/05/96 SALBUTAMOL                   INH 100.00             28      1        -




















Allergy/Int: AR - penicillamine
    Date     Formulary name           Frm Strngth Dosage     Days   Qty op Rp Is P/N
```

Figure 30   The therapy add (TA) screen in Vamp

The main difference between this and other templating systems is that freehand uses an entirely separate dictionary of terms for the recording of data. This dictionary is referred to as the 'freehand line dictionary', and is quite limited in nature, containing between 300 and 400 items. Users cannot currently add to it.

Some freehand items are related to the same items on the PD screen but beyond this the system (apart from sharing a common patient list) is quite separate. This must be borne in mind when planning its implementation On the plus side, quite a lot of user customisation is possible and it is easy to modify the lists of choices that apply to freehand lines.

Setting up a freehand template or modifying an existing one is also quite straightforward at a basic level, i.e. it is quite easy to alter/add/remove lines from a freehand template, but somewhat more difficult to alter the way in which data from other parts of the system is displayed, e.g. medical history, item repeats, etc.

Figure 31 shows an asthma freehand template.

Macros

Before moving on to consider the reporting options in Vamp, it is important to mention one feature that does not appear as a native feature of either of the two other major systems, namely 'macros'.

A macro is an automated sequence of keystrokes that can be 'played back' by pressing a particular key combination. They are frequently used in word processing programs to automate repetitive tasks, but Vamp has always had a macro facility as standard. (Other terminal-based systems can use the built in macro facilities of the terminals to implement something similar, but in general this is less successful.)

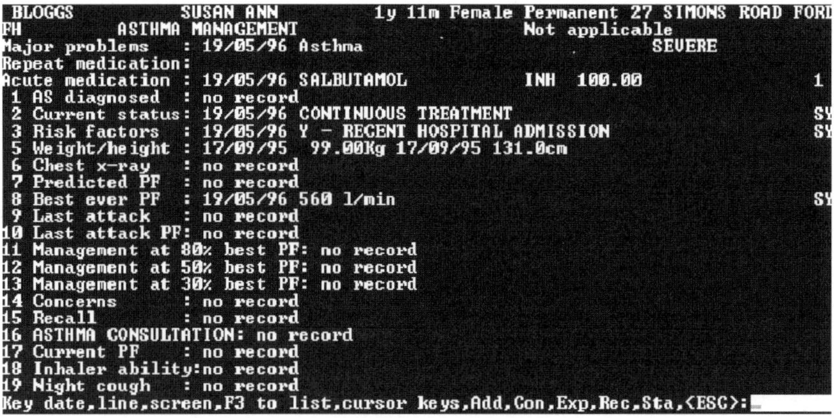

```
BLOGGS         SUSAN ANN            1y 11m Female Permanent 27 SIMONS ROAD FORD
PH        ASTHMA MANAGEMENT                        Not applicable
Major problems    : 19/05/96 Asthma                           SEVERE
Repeat medication:
Acute medication  : 19/05/96 SALBUTAMOL            INH  100.00             1
 1 AS diagnosed   : no record
 2 Current status : 19/05/96 CONTINUOUS TREATMENT                          SY
 3 Risk factors   : 19/05/96 Y - RECENT HOSPITAL ADMISSION                 SY
 5 Weight/height  : 17/09/95    99.00Kg 17/09/95 131.0cm
 6 Chest x-ray    : no record
 7 Predicted PF   : no record
 8 Best ever PF   : 19/05/96 560 l/min                                     SY
 9 Last attack    : no record
10 Last attack PF : no record
11 Management at 80% best PF: no record
12 Management at 50% best PF: no record
13 Management at 30% best PF: no record
14 Concerns       : no record
15 Recall         : no record
16 ASTHMA CONSULTATION: no record
17 Current PF     : no record
18 Inhaler ability:no record
19 Night cough    : no record
Key date,line,screen,F3 to list,cursor keys,Add,Con,Exp,Rec,Sta,<ESC>:
```

Figure 31   The freehand asthma screen

By setting up macros, users can automatically enter an item into the patient's medical history (HA) set up a prescription (TA) and print it (TP). In this way 40 or 50 keystrokes can be reduced to three.

This technique is only really useful for those things that routinely occur in a standard way. As an example, a one off occurrence of cystitis treated with trimethoprim could be handled this way. If the entry required a unique free-text comment, it could not. Further, this technique is only truly useful where a certain diagnosis invariably leads to a particular drug being prescribed.

Some practices only use macros to speed up the input of drugs and do not use them at all for medical history items. Many practices use them to speed up the issue of 'flu jabs, for example.

Standard Reports/Practice Analysis

Vamp is well equipped, with a relatively large number of standard reports to cover much of the routine reporting required of the practice.

These exist in two separate areas:

- Vamp reporter
- Practice analysis

These two areas are quite separate, with practice analysis being a transaction available within the main Vamp system and reporter being an entirely separate program available from the Vamp start-up menu before entering Vamp Medical.

Practice analysis covers such items as cytology and immunisations, and the now unnecessary (but useful) health-promotion reports. Vamp reporter is a fully fledged application in its own right providing a large number of standard reports, covering areas like patient contact rates, computer usage and prescribing habits. It also provides a large number of detailed reports on basic health data.

Most of these reports just require the input of a few items of data, such as a date range to run and, as such, can be highly effective in giving members of the practice access to the data, even when they are not clear about using the report generator. Figure 32 shows a referral report being set up.

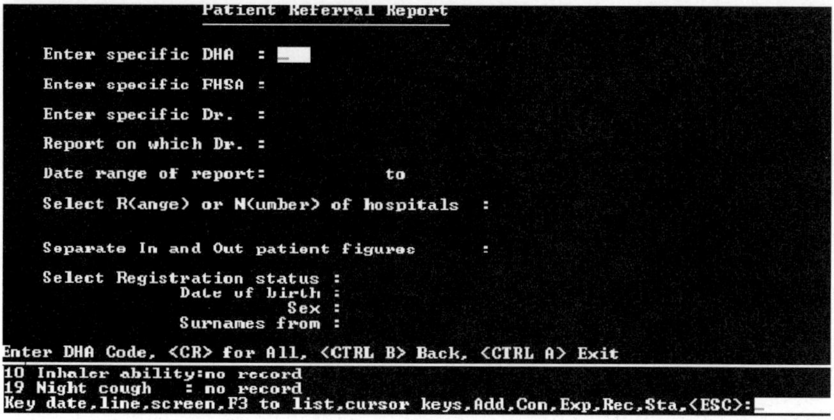

Figure 32 Setting up a referral report in Vamp

Report Generator and Freehand Reports

Vamp has two report generators for non-standard reports: one for freehand and one for all other data contained in the system. It is also the case that each of these systems works in a different way, necessitating extra familiarisation for those practices wishing to get the best out of it. We will look at the 'standard' report generator first.

Using the Vamp transaction SR brings up the main search menu as shown in Figure 33.

The VAMP Medical System

```
Search Menu

1  Registration
2  Epidemiology
3  Drug
4  Medical History
5  Prevention options
6  FreeHand Searches
7  Save/Print last search
8  Process Groups
9  Process Saved Searches

Select option    ▪

<CR> to return to Transaction prompt
```

Figure 33 The main search menu in Vamp

Notice that the freehand report generator is started from this menu but after this it works in a different way.

In some ways Vamp does not have a report generator in the true sense, as although all the report types on this menu (except freehand) share common features, each is different depending on the item(s) being reported. Most of the search types shown lead initially to a screen similar to the one in Figure 34, which is the one used for searching OXMIS or Read codes.

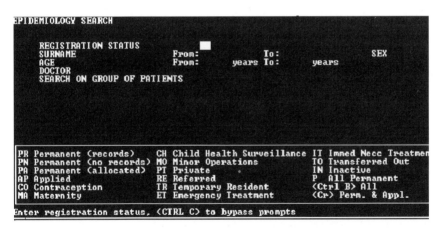

Figure 34 The Vamp epidemiology search screen

After filling in the default information for this search (epidemiology) the system then prompts for an OXMIS or Read code or codes. Codes can be combined (logical AND, OR and NOT) and OXMIS codes can be mixed with Read codes. This makes the reporting flexible, but output is restricted to a list of selected patients' names and addresses or the saving of a group for further processing.

The other types of search on the main search menu are mostly self-explanatory. Prevention options allow searching of basic health data as stored on the prevention screen. Medical history searches allow searching on all the other details of medical record entries (history), including the priority number episode, GP, etc.

The last two items on the search menu refer to groups. This is another little-used (but very useful) feature of the system which allows the patients found, as a result of a search, to be added in various ways or subtracted from another group. In this way complex searches can gradually be built up, accessing data in all parts of the Vamp system. It should, perhaps, be said that this process could take some time to complete!

Freehand Searches

Freehand searches and reports apply to the data stored in freehand templates and work in a completely different way to normal Vamp searches. Basically, they allow all aspects of a particular freehand line (defined earlier) to be reported. In freehand, as well as being able to define a search to isolate a group of patients, a report format can also be specified showing the data to be output. Although the integration of the freehand report generator with the rest of the Vamp system is not strong, freehand reports will accept groups derived from other searches as the input data, and can save the output of a freehand search to a group. Figure 35 shows a freehand search for the line FH of ischaemic heart disease.

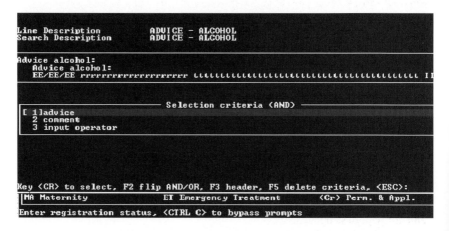

Figure 35   The Vamp freehand search screen

All in all, freehand adds a major dimension to the scope and functionality of the Vamp medical system. Although it is essentially a separate system sharing a common patient base, it is well worth developing skills in its use as a number of tasks are either very difficult or impossible without it.

Closing Summary

Vamp is a difficult system to sum up. It is probably true to say that it is idiosyncratic in its user interface and limited in terms of its clinical record structure, but most users of this system like it and find it easy to use.

Until the release of the latest major upgrade to this system, it was easy to think that VAMP would quietly let it die in favour of Vamp Vision, but now that it is able to use Read codes and can accept unlimited text in the clinical record, the situation seems to have changed.

Vamp Medical, despite its limitations, might well prove to be the best choice for practices where the degree of general practitioner involvement is always going to be limited. It is quite capable of storing and reporting a wide variety of clinical and non-clinical information, and is a good starting point for a practice which has previously been uncomputerised.

At a glance: VAMP Medical

Strengths	Features	Ratings (on a scale of 1–10)
Very easy to use with all the basic facilities required for limited data entry.	Administration/ registration data	✓✓✓✓✓
	Consultation data	✓✓✓
Powerful macro feature allows common tasks to be automated.	Reporting	✓✓✓✓✓✓
	Templates	✓✓✓✓
	Integration	✓
Most recent versions are Read (rather than OXMIS) coded and have unlimited free text.	Look and feel	✓✓✓
	Costs	✓✓✓✓
	Support	✓✓✓✓✓✓✓
Competent (and basic) reporting.	Overall	✓✓✓✓

Weaknesses
A mixture of different types of data-entry screen, but not suitable for paperless operation.
Limited functionality.
Rather old fashioned when compared with its rivals.

8
Other Systems

Opening Summary

This chapter discusses a number of systems from different suppliers as well as covering the two major new Windows-based systems from Vamp and AAH Meditel.

Introduction

The aim of this chapter is to describe briefly a number of the other systems commonly in use and to include basic details of the two major new Windows-based systems from AAH Meditel and Vamp. These system are broadly representative of those available from suppliers other than the 'big three'.

The systems that will be covered in this chapter are:

- Vamp Vision
- AAH Meditel System 6000
- Ambridge
- Torex Premiere
- Amsys
- Seetec

Vamp Vision

The Vamp Vision system is one of the new generation of general practice systems to be written to utilise the Windows GUI. The Vision system can be supplied as a turnkey system with all software and hardware supplied by Vamp. Alternatively, practices can acquire most of their hardware from third parties and buy just the software and some critical elements of the hardware from Vamp. This will almost certainly reduce initial costs to some extent, but may well lead to increased difficulties for the practice if the source of a particular problem it not clear.

The system is LAN based and requires a high-specification server in order to run at an adequate speed. The workstations must also be of a high specification, both in terms of their processor and their RAM.

Entry into each module of the system is from push buttons on a menu. Within each module standard menus and toolbars allow different functions to be carried out. The system is extremely powerful but this means that it can be confusing to use at first. The screen shots shown are from v. 1.15 and are slightly different in the latest version.

Registration

The registration module is straightforward in operation and contains a number of useful features. When registering a new patient, screens are stepped through in a logical order. The concept of families is supported. When adding new patients, missing data is highlighted in red. Mandatory data cannot be skipped, although in some cases, after a warning, data can be omitted. This can be confusing. The system does not favour the use of computer numbers but allows existing patients to be selected by a range of factors including DOB, surname (default), road name, postcode, etc. The status of existing patients can easily be changed. Several of the fields in the registration area contain pop-ups from which a response can be selected. This is quick and convenient in use. However, most of the pop-ups are not user-definable.

Patient Data

The consultation manager in Vision is a complex piece of software in its own right. It is accessed via the appropriate button on the main menu. There are many default options which can be set within consultation manager, such as whether a new consultation is started when a patient is selected and what data from the record is initially available. Many options concerning the display of information can also be set.

There are two basic views plus a summary screen. The first of these is the medical record overview (Figure 36). Data is grouped into the headings shown on the left-hand side of the screen, with a numerical indication of how many items exist in a particular category. Double clicking an item with the mouse, e.g. consultations, displays summary data for consultations on the right of the screen. Double clicking a particular item then displays more detail in a window that opens at the bottom right of the screen.

Once a consultation has been started, data can be added. This can be done in the screen in Figure 36 by using the menu system or by using a right mouse click and the Add option. Alternatively, the consultation manager screen can be used (Figure 37).

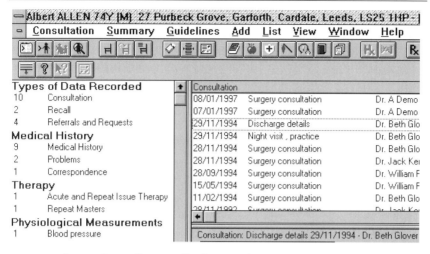

Figure 36 The medical overview screen in Vision

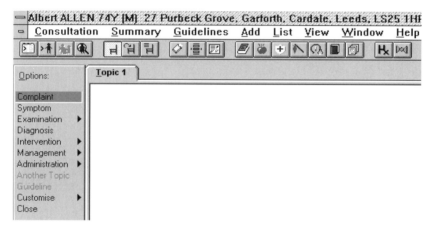

Figure 37 The consultation manager screen

Data can be added to this screen according to the categories that appear on the left of the screenshot. The system uses the concept of problems. Instead, items are grouped under problems retrospectively, which, although it seems long-winded, works well in practice.

One of the major benefits of this system is its ability to use a Read code formulary rather than the full Read code system. This has the advantage that new users do not need to be exposed to the full Read code dictionary, but instead can select from a much smaller dictionary defined by the practice.

The system is equipped with a large number of forms for the recording of common information for basic health, asthma, etc but additionally has a templating system (referred to as guidelines) which again is supplied with several usable templates which can be modified by the practice. The system allows screen lists to be displayed under general headings that can then be expanded into detailed entries. Figure 38 shows a diabetic guideline in use, with the Examination entries expanded. Entries can be added by right clicking on the relevant line.

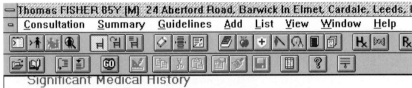

Figure 38   The Vamp Vision diabetic management screen

For those GPs who initially do not wish to use the full consultation manager facilities, historical data can be entered using a screen not unlike the history screen in the old Vamp Medical system. Here single-dated Read-coded entries can be made (even using the priority number system from the old system).

As with other modern systems, prescribing is carried out as an integral part of the consultation, with all the normal facilities present, such as generic substitution, etc. Acutes and repeats are handled in separate screens but in a very similar manner.

Both referrals and referral letters can be generated by the system with the word processing done in a cut-down version of Microsoft Word, or optionally in Word itself. Full mailmerge facilities are also present.

Vamp was one of the first suppliers to operate effective GP–HA links, and Vision uses much the same system as the older Vamp Medical system, but with more integrated pathology links. Fully Read-coded data can be transmitted directly to the practice and incorporated in the patient record in much the same way as if data input had been done at the practice.

Reporting

Vamp Vision is equipped with comprehensive search and reporting facilities. These are accessed via the appropriate button on the main menu. An array of preconfigured reports is supplied, including individual patient reports as well as target and referral reports, etc. More general searches are also available. The search generator screen is shown in Figure 39.

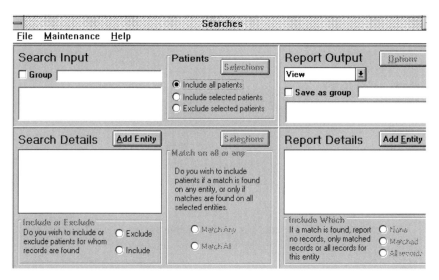

Figure 39   The Vamp search screen

Searches can be made on a wide variety of parameters and all the normal features are present. A new search is created by first selecting the input. This can be based on the results of a previous search (group) or on registration parameters of patients. The actual search conditions are entered under 'Search Details' and can include all the different types of data present, such as Read codes or prescriptions. Multiple conditions can be stated and free text can be searched if desired. Read-coded searches can be either for a specific code or can include all sub-codes. The detail of clinical entries can also be fully searched. Individual searches are all OR or all AND. By this multiple criteria either all have to be true to select patients or any can be true. In order to handle a mixed situation (x OR y AND z) a search must be done, saved as a group, and then used as the input to the second search.

Once a search has been done, there is a great degree of flexibility in relation to how the information held on these patients can be output. Basically, most data that is recorded can be included for the selected patients. There are various types of output report format, but these depend to some extent on the type of information being sought. Currently, output formats are not user-definable. It is possible to export to an ASCII file or a spreadsheet. Interestingly, if a search is output to the screen it appears as a list of patients. Double-clicking a patient then brings up the selected clinical entries for that patient. This is a very useful feature for quick searches of limited groups of individuals.

Conclusions

Vamp Vision is much more flexible and modern than most of the other general practice systems available. It has obviously been the subject of a great deal of development. As a consequence of its flexibility it is somewhat difficult to come to grips with at first, but perseverance is worthwhile.

The Read code formulary is an obvious improvement, which can lead to the much more effective and quicker use of Read codes, especially in those practices previously not using them at all. The search facilities within Vision are very powerful.

The review given here is based on version 1.15, but as the book went to press a new version (2.0) was starting to be distributed to VAMP practices. This version solves many of the initial minor criticisms of the system. In particular, it introduces full integration of the Multilex drug dictionary (contraindications and interactions are now fully supported) and the ability to add data directly to a problem. Other major changes include a new consultation screen with the ability to show the chronological sequence of a problem (timelines) as well as improved interface features and many new reports. The guidelines feature is now very powerful with prescribing available from within a guideline.

Vamp Vision is a comprehensive system that currently suits those practices that are keen to enter clinical data in the consultation and then be in a position to be able to analyse it. It is possibly less well suited to those who enter little clinical data, as it would be overly complex in these situations.

Other Systems 113

At a glance: **VAMP Vision**

Strengths	Features	Ratings (on a scale of 1–10)
Powerful and up-to-date system for practices who wish to make significant clinical use of their system.	Administration/ registration data	✓✓✓✓✓✓✓
	Consultation data	✓✓✓✓✓✓✓✓
	Reporting	✓✓✓✓✓✓✓✓
Well-developed Read code formulary system which works well.	Templates	✓✓✓✓✓✓✓
	Integration	✓✓✓✓✓✓✓✓
Good reporting system.	Look and feel	✓✓✓✓✓✓✓✓
Latest version significantly improved, particularly in consultation.	Costs	✓✓✓✓
	Support	✓✓✓✓✓✓✓
	Overall	✓✓✓✓✓✓✓
Worthy competition for EMIS and AAH Meditel.		

Weaknesses

Requires powerful hardware and can be confusing initially owing to the range of options.

Only loosely related to Vamp Medical in a few respects.

AAH Meditel System 6000

System 6000 is AAH Meditel's new Windows-based system enjoying the same relationship to the 'old' system (System 5) that Vamp Vision has to Vamp Medical. The system, although Windows based, uses a UNIX server on the desktop to do all of the main work, and can be cited as an example of a *client/server* system. This has a number of important consequences, not the least of which is that practices with existing AAH Meditel systems can, for the time being, continue to make use of dumb terminals in undemanding situations (i.e. reception). They can use the full Windows-based client program in consulting rooms and other locations where the sophistication and power of the Windows interface can be fully utilised.

Again in contrast to Vision (which can be regarded as an entirely new program), 6000 is more of an evolution from the existing System 5. This evolution makes it easy for existing AAH Meditel users to use the system immediately as, for example, the function key assignments are the same in both systems.

Registration

The registration screen in System 6000 is shown in Figure 40.

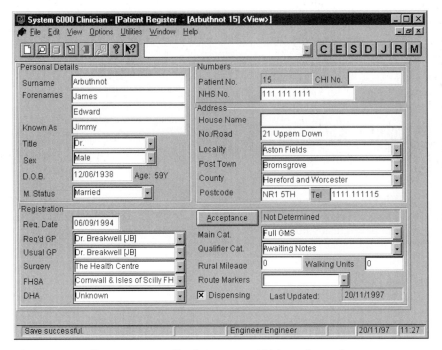

Figure 40 The AAH Meditel System 6000 registration screen

Adding a patient in System 6000 is, in many respects, similar to the procedure in System 5. Once a patient has been selected, the name appears on the file menu, making it easy to reselect them if desired. This feature is also present in Vision, although here the last nine patients are listed. As would be expected, most of the details are added from drop-down menus (not user definable). The registration screen shown in the screenshot can be thought of as a summary screen with each section having further screens 'below' it. Most of the information in these further screens below it is optional (i.e. hospital and other contact addresses). The system is able to build up a patient address dictionary, making the subsequent addition of patients with similar addresses easier. There is also a new system for grouping patients into families, which is more sophisticated than the facility built into System 5. Patients can be identified on the basis of 13 different parameters, and the use of similar function keys as in System 5 ensures that AAH Meditel practices who upgrade will have a head start. Normal Windows mouse/menu systems can, of course, also be used.

Patient Data

The clinical data parts of the AAH Meditel system are all new, but a lot of the powerful problem-oriented features of the old system have been retained. As with Vamp Vision there are a number of different screens in which to view clinical information. Figure 41 shows the summary view with its four windows and registration data at the top of the screen. Note particularly the buttons C, E, S, D, etc in the top part of the screenshot. These are similar to the single-letter options in System 5 and allow quick movement to another view of the data (i.e. C for Current, etc).

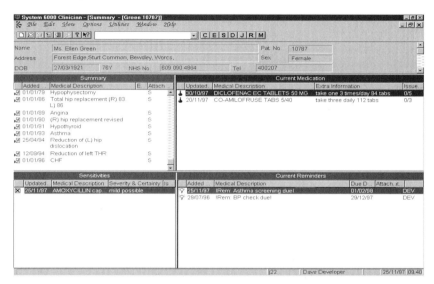

Figure 41   The AAH Meditel System 6000 summary screen

The system is highly user configurable (again like Vision) in that the default opening screen can be set up so that information is displayed in a form suitable for that particular user. There are also many useful warnings and prompts, such as a warning if a temporary resident is out of date.

As would be expected, data can be added in any of the available clinical screens, but it is best (again following the model established with System 5) if it is entered via the current problems screen. In Figure 42, the current screen is shown with asthma screening highlighted. All the entries related to this problem are shown on the right-hand side of the screen.

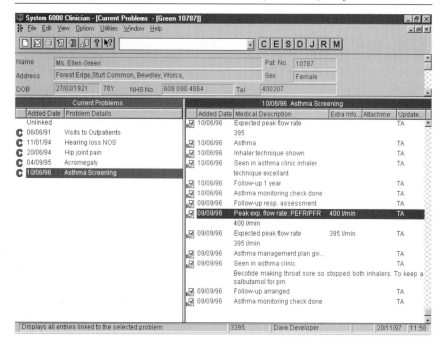

Figure 42 The AAH Meditel System 6000 current screen

One very useful new feature is the ability to put in end dates for the range of clinical data. This neatly side-steps one of the problems of Read coding where a patient has two mutually exclusive conditions at different times (i.e. IDDM/NIDDM).

Templates and protocols are handled via a development of the SOPHIE system which first appeared in System 5, but it is much more sophisticated in the new program. An example of this is the ability of SOPHIE to run automatically in the background (Watchdogs) enforcing practice protocols. It could be set up automatically to prompt for a blood-pressure reading on a patient with a certain Read-coded diagnosis, i.e. hypertension – if a reading had not been entered within a certain period. This is in contrast to the older system where the SOPHIE protocol would have to 'run' specifically for this patient in order to make this warning appear.

The process of creating protocol templates has also been made very much easier with the addition of a Windows-type 'Wizard' to guide the user through the process step by step. As has recently become the case with System 5, advice sheets can be dispensed to patients as part of the process. Figure 43 shows a SOPHIE template being used for geriatric surveillance.

Other Systems 117

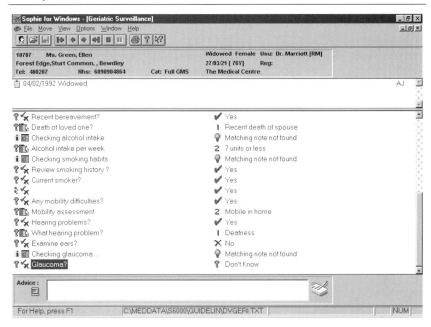

Figure 43 The AAH Meditel System 6000 SOPHIE protocol

The medication module is significantly enhanced over the one that appeared in System 5 and takes full advantage of the Windows environment, although the use of the same function keys again aids practices when upgrading from System 5. The sensitivities feature is much enhanced and medication is more explicitly linked to a related problem (i.e. repeats can be 'reauthorised' either globally or just for the medication relating to a particular problem). The drug formulary is also enhanced and selections can be applied globally or individually.

Two novel features that apply to System 6000 are the ability to store pictures and the provision of a free-text note system. Pictures can be stored as part of the patient record and this means that not only can the output of various diagnostic tests be stored, but also that freehand sketches can also be inserted; for example, showing the position of a suspect breast lump. The notepad system is interesting in that it is a free-text window that can contain *ad hoc* data about the patient in rather the same way as attaching a yellow sticky 'Post-it' note to the manual records. Although not linked to the main structure of the patients record, it does also display reminders from the record. Finally, all the normal facilities to write referral letters exist and AAH Meditel say that any Windows-based word processor can be used with the system.

Reporting

A wide variety of predefined searches and reports (several hundred) are supplied with the system, but customised reporting is also catered for with the inclusion of a sophisticated query generator. The main screen of this is shown in Figure 44.

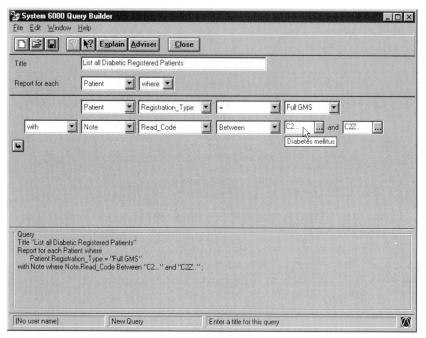

Figure 44 The AAH Meditel System 6000 query builder

As can be seen from the screenshot, the building-up of queries is fairly self-explanatory, with choices being made from drop-down lists. Multiple criteria are catered for, and as the criteria of the report are built up, the query itself is listed at the bottom of the screen.

As well as queries (searches), there are a large number of report formats that can be applied to them to extract the desired information for the selected patients. In addition, the final output can be saved in a format suitable for use in a stand-alone spreadsheet package (ASCII and spreadsheet).

Conclusions

The AAH Meditel System 6000 is a worthy rival to the other major Windows-based system on the market, namely VAMP Vision. Clearly, the use of the Windows interface makes this program superficially

Other Systems 119

resemble VAMP Vision, but System 6000 is much more of a development of System 5 than Vision is of Vamp Medical, making it particularly attractive as an upgrade option to current System 5 users. Although the two programs are somewhat similar in their range of features, a major strength of the AAH Meditel system is the very strong problem orientation of the clinical record. Another major difference between the two is the choice of the underlying operating system. System 6000 is based on a UNIX server which, although a more complex technical solution, does allow a system to retain some dumb terminals.

At a glance: AAH Meditel System 6000

Strengths	Features	Ratings (on a scale of 1–10)
The other major new Windows-based system. The years of development seem to have paid off with this very competent successor to System 5. Similar functionality to Vision but with strong problem orientation.	Administration/ registration data Consultation data Reporting Templates Integration Look and feel Costs Support Overall	✔✔✔✔✔✔✔✔ ✔✔✔✔✔✔✔✔✔ ✔✔✔✔✔✔✔ ✔✔✔✔✔ ✔✔✔✔✔✔✔✔✔ ✔✔✔✔✔✔✔✔✔ ✔✔✔✔✔ ✔✔✔✔✔✔✔ ✔✔✔✔✔✔✔

Weaknesses
SOPHIE not as easy to use as it could be. Too early in the release cycle to comment on stability.

The Torex GP Manager System (Previously Ambridge)

This system, ranks in the top five systems, with several hundred sites using it. The system described here (v. 2.3) is text based. A major upgrade (GP Manager, v. 3) is soon to appear and will be RFA 4 accredited (Requirements for Accreditation, v. 4). Torex have recently introduced a Windows-based system called Torex Premiere which appeared in mid-1998 and is briefly reviewed later in this chapter.

GP Manager is UNIX based and can be described as a multi-user configuration with a central computer attached to dumb terminals. In many practices the screens are Windows PCs running a terminal-emulator program.

The system is text based and navigation is carried out by using two letter codes to open particular modules in the same manner as AAH

Meditel and others. These codes run to three screen pages, indicating the number of available modules. It is also possible to navigate around the screens using the up and down arrow keys.

Registration Data

The registration screen in GP Manager is conventional and supports all the normal data items. The concept of 'families' is supported as is partial support for an address dictionary. As with a number of other systems, a distinction is made between the registered GP and the one usually seen here – termed the 'caring' GP. As GP Manager supports registration (and IOS) links, some of the fields on the registration screen are mandatory. Some of the picking lists used are user-amendable. Figure 45 shows the registration screen.

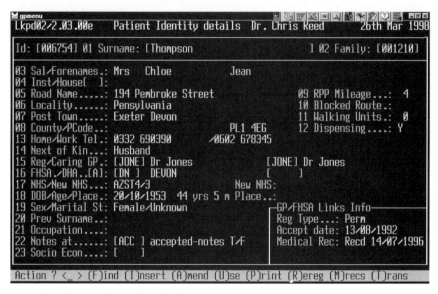

Figure 45   The registration screen in GP Manager

Clinical Data

Prescribing is not integrated with the entry of other data in the same way as it is in EMIS and AAH Meditel, but is accessed via a separate screen. The system uses a Read-coded drug dictionary and is conventional in most respects. It is possible with this system to by-pass the drug dictionary entirely and enter the required drug in free text, but this is not to be recommended as searching on items entered in this way is not possible.

The main area for the entry of clinical information is the MR (Medical Records) module. This is conventional in layout, resembling the HA screen in Vamp somewhat, but additionally with a degree of structure possible in the record. Entries can be made directly to this screen (episodes) or as notes attached to existing episodes (encounters). There are a number of options for changing the appearance of the MR screen. A particular entry can comprise a date, type (user defined if appropriate via a set-up option) and a Read code, followed by user ID (defaults to the logged-on user), department (GPs, nurses, etc), time and a numeric value for the priority of the encounter (1–9). Free text can be entered next to Read-coded entries, or as an alternative to Read codes. Up to six lines of data constitute a single entry, allowing detailed recording of encounters.

Read codes are entered via the appropriate rubric or by direct entry of the Read code. Although all the normal facilities exist, it is necessary to use the F1 function key to select a Read code that is not at the bottom of the hierarchy. In practice, this different action (normally pressing return selects the term) can be a little off-putting, particularly if a significant number of higher level terms are in use.

The templates in GP Manager are fully user definable and, while not as easy to set up as, say, EMIS or Vamp Medical, are nevertheless well within the abilities of most practices. Items that are to be added to templates have to be predefined and normally consist of a Read code and some extra data field, such as a numeric value or free text. The practice can also define a short code (e.g. BP for blood pressure) which can be linked to the Read code.

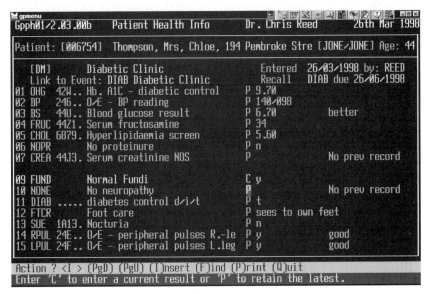

Figure 46   The health information screen in GP Manager

Searches

Searching in GP Manager is comprehensive, both searches and reports being user definable, with a number of standard reports available separately. As well as producing reports, the results of searches can be used to create mail-merge letters in conjunction with the simple word processor mentioned in the previous section. It should be said, however, that the methods of setting up searches and reports, while powerful and flexible, are at first sight rather complex involving the use of several of the program modules. In addition, many practices may take some time to come to grips with the required techniques. Figure 47 shows an extract criteria being constructed.

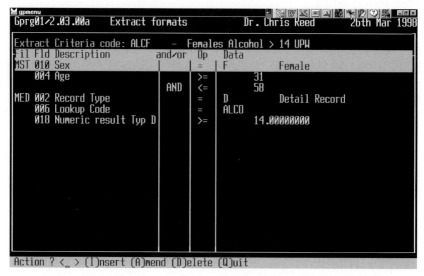

Figure 47 Extract criteria in GP Manager reporting

Conclusions

GP Manager is a comprehensive clinical system that can be supplied with a number of other programs such as GP Ledger, GP Payroll etc. In general look and feel it most resembles AAH Meditel System 5 (probably due to the use of essentially the same operating system) but its templates are much easier to set up (but less powerful).

This trade of ease-of-use versus sophistication means that this system is probably best suited to those practices who have moderate plans for the entry of clinical data. In this situation the ease with which the system can be mastered would be an advantage. Additionally, qualitative research amongst users showed that GP Manager users were generally the most satisfied with the service they received from the company.

At a glance: GP Manager

Strengths	Features	Ratings (on a scale of 1–10)
A functional, if basic, UNIX-based system with the major elements needed by all but paperless practices.	Administration/ registration data	✓✓✓✓✓
	Consultation data	✓✓✓
	Reporting	✓✓✓✓
It has a degree of problem orientation.	Templates	✓✓✓✓
	Integration	✓✓
Liked by its users and considered good value for money.	Look and feel	✓✓✓✓
	Costs	✓✓✓✓✓✓
Easy to use (apart from reports).	Support	✓✓✓✓✓✓✓✓
	Overall	✓✓✓✓✓

Weaknesses
Searches can be complex to set up.
Problem orientation and clinical record are less sophisticated than EMIS or AAH Meditel.

The Torex Premiere System

This system, which has only recently become generally available, is notable because it is another full Windows system. The version reviewed is a slightly earlier version than that released to practices. The following details are necessarily brief owing to the fact that at the time of writing there were few practices using the system. However, a significant number of practices plan to change to this system.

The system can be supplied with either a Windows NT-based server or a UNIX server and can (like System 6000) support a mixture of dumb terminals and Windows PCs. Clearly there are some differences between the look of the program in these two different environments, but the basic functionality remains the same. In contrast to other products, Torex Premiere owes little to the older products from the same company. It is an entirely new product in terms of functionality and concept, having little in common with the Torex non-Windows products, other than similar data tables.

Registration

The registration screen in Torex Premiere is shown in Figure 48. This is the first of a number of screens used to register a patient, and is similar to other programs in terms of the fields required. Various methods of selecting patients exist, e.g. on surname, ID, forename, address, etc with combinations of fields being accepted.

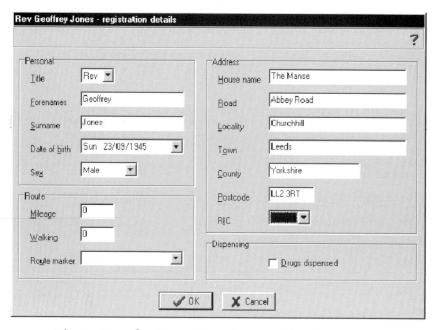

Figure 48   The Torex Premiere registration screen

Patient Data

One of the benefits of Torex Premiere is that it is fairly simple to use, with most data entry being carried out from a single type of screen. Figure 49 shows the main patient summary screen – one of a number of summary views provided. Others include clinical notes – an electronic chronological representation of all of the data, repeats and health-promotion data.

As with other Windows-based systems, there are a variety of ways of inputting data into the system from this screen. These include using keyboard shortcuts, the menu system or clicking on buttons on the toolbar. Data entry is categorised into a number of sections, such as morbidity, prescription, referrals, etc. Basic measurements are also handled in this way with menu items existing for information such as height and weight. Problems are supported within the system and a morbidity can be made into a problem by entering a start date for it. Data can be added to existing problems.

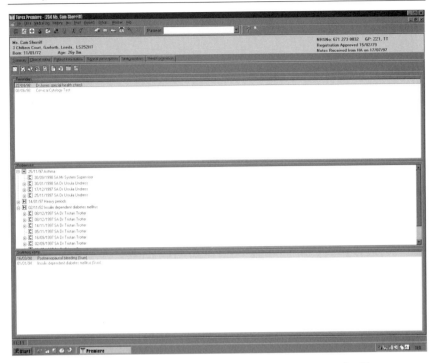

Figure 49 The main patient summary screen in Torex Premiere

Read codes are added to the system via a pop-up dialogue box and are entered by typing in a part of the Read code rubric or a user-defined synonym. It is particularly easy to add synonyms to the system. Various qualifiers to Read coded data can be entered if desired, e.g. status – first, new or ongoing, laterality – left, right, etc and certainty – clinical, definite, etc. Figure 50 shows asthma being entered into a patient's record.

Drugs are added to the patient record in a similar fashion to Read codes. The BNF hierarchy can be browsed and practice formularies are supported. All the normal interactions/contraindications are also shown. Generic substitution of a drug is carried out using a button on the prescribing screen. User-defined short codes can be added, either individually or by the practice as a whole, to make the access to particular drugs easier. The system supports a degree of learning ability promoting often used drugs to the top of picking lists in much the same way as EMIS.

The templating system in Torex Premiere is called ISIS. A number of templates are supplied and new ones can be created by users. The system works by presenting the user with a sequence of dialog boxes, one for each data item to be captured. These items are then added to the patient record in the same way as if they had been entered individually.

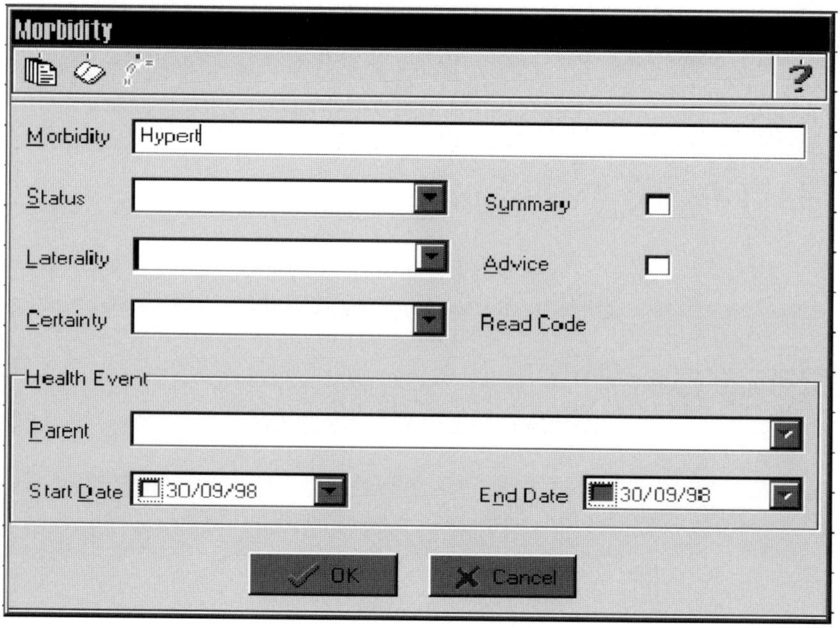

Figure 50 Adding a Read-coded morbidity to Torex Premiere

Reporting

A number of standard reports exist within the system for such items as referrals, targets, etc. There is also a search generator which will search on any data entered into the system.

The search engine is a reasonable compromise between ease of use and power, with single criteria searches being easy to set up. Facilities exist for multi-parameter searches, but these require more thought. It would appear that every field in the system can be searched, but this comprehensive ability means that finding the required field to be searched can be confusing as there is a very long list of available fields. Figure 51 shows a simple asthma search being constructed.

Having completed a search, the resulting group of patients is referred to as a 'hitlist'. This group of patients may then be printed or viewed to screen with or without selected clinical and/or registration data. Fully user-defined output reports are not currently available, but the needs of a majority of users will be catered for with the list of preset options. There is, however, the facility to export most clinical data to other programs.

Other Systems 127

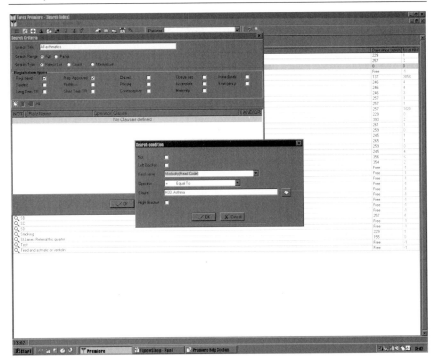

Figure 51 The Torex Premiere search screen

Conclusions

The Torex Premiere system is a difficult system to categorise. Ultimately it lacks the sophistication of products like AAH Meditel System 6000 and Vamp Vision, but, on the other hand, it is very easy to use. It also has more functionality than most non-Windows systems, particularly in its implementation of problems which, like AAH System 6000, involve the use of start and end dates. The templating system ISIS is functional, although not as powerful as in other systems. The reporting is weaker than that in, for example, Vision, but adequate for most needs. An appointment system is available, although this has not been reviewed.

Torex Premiere may well have been designed from the outset with ease of use as the main priority, and in this way the system will be attractive to those practices who want a Windows system but who want to be able to get to grips with it easily. It should also be borne in mind that this product is at the very start of its development cycle and the final version released to practices may include further features.

In October 1998 Torex PLC acquired Hollowbrook Computer Services Ltd, significantly increasing their share of the GP market and making them a rival to Meditel for the number three position.

At a glance:	**The Torex Premiere System**	
Strengths	**Features**	**Ratings** (on a scale of 1–10)
Another new Windows-based system from Torex should fill a gap in the market for practices who want a straightforward easy-to-use Windows system. Only just released, so should only get better.	Administration/ registration data	✔✔✔✔✔✔
	Consultation data	✔✔✔✔✔✔✔✔
	Reporting	✔✔✔✔✔✔✔
	Templates	✔✔✔✔✔✔
	Integration	✔✔✔✔✔✔✔✔
	Look and feel	✔✔✔✔✔✔✔
	Costs ⎱ Support ⎰	Insufficient data available to form a judgement
	Overall	✔✔✔✔✔✔✔
Weaknesses		
A bit weak on reporting – no fully user-defined reports and still some rough edges in the version reviewed. Some actions non-intuitive		

Amsys

Amsys is one of the systems produced by LK Global. This company also supports the Genisyst clinical and fundholding systems and has also recently introduced a Windows-based clinical program. LK Global collectively is also in the top six in terms of numbers of sites, with the majority of sites currently using the software reviewed here, often in conjunction with Genisyst fundholding software.

The Amsys software is DOS based and a LAN (normally Novell) is employed. The software is written using the Advanced Revelation Database Management System (a database management system (DBMS) that provides all of the basic database functionality that is necessary), although this is almost incidental to users. The system employs five-digit Read codes and is menu driven with the cursor keys or a highlighted letter being used to select menu items. The main menu is shown in Figure 52.

Registration

As with GP Manager, the registration screen in Amsys is entirely conventional. Patients are not referred to by a computer-generated number but by a key generated as a combination of their initials and their date of birth. Most of the choices on the registration screen are

Other Systems

entered by selecting from predefined pop-up menus. There are no self-building address dictionaries. Once the first stage of adding a new patient has been confirmed it is difficult to cancel the patient. A facility exists to add several members of the same family at the same time.

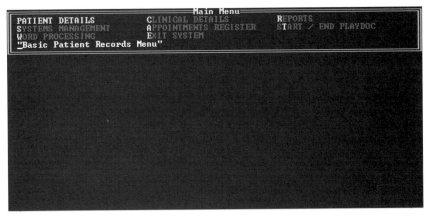

Figure 52 The Amsys menu system

Patient Data

There are several areas within Amsys where patients' clinical data can be added. These include consultations, significant medical history, disease log, a number of clinics, etc. It must be borne in mind that all of these areas are separate, and while it is possible to add data semi-automatically from, say, a consultation to the significant medical history, searching a particular Read code only includes entries in specified areas. In this way the system differs from others such as AAH Meditel, EMIS and Vamp Vision. Entry of data can normally be Read coded or free text. Figure 53 shows the consultation screen in Amsys.

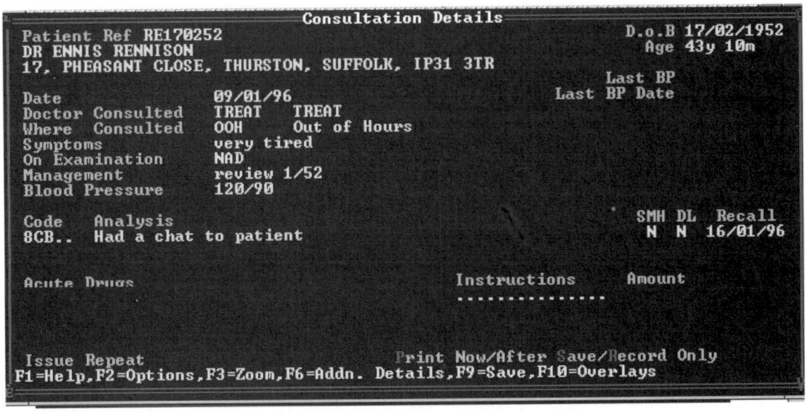

Figure 53 Adding a consultation in Amsys

Both Read-coded data and acute drugs can be added to this screen. Any Read-coded data entered can also be automatically copied to the significant medical history and disease log by putting Y (Yes) in the appropriate fields. It is easy (by design) to cancel the coded entry of data in the Read-code area and in the prescription of drugs, and if this is done free text data can then be added at will. While this gives the system a certain flexibility at the point of data entry, it could lead to difficulties in extracting data later. For similar reasons it is important to decide precisely what data is included in the SMH and DL areas.

The Read-code browsing facilities are adequate, with Read codes being directly accessible by their rubrics or the actual codes themselves. Codes can easily be selected at any particular level and the entry of Read-coded data is quick.

Drugs are entered from the Philex drug dictionary and, apart from being able to override the dictionary and enter anything, this aspect is generally conventional. Drug interactions are displayed, if relevant. Swapping to a generic form of a drug (and vice versa) is also supported using a function key combination.

Referrals are entered via a special screen and, in addition, Read-coded data can be added to the details of the referral in a similar fashion to consultations.

As well as a number of predefined screens for clinics, such as asthma and diabetes (which cannot be altered by the users), there is a facility by which simple user-defined templates can be made. This facility, although not as developed as in some other systems, is nevertheless useful.

Searches

As with other systems, there are a large number of predefined reports available within the system covering all the usual areas. In addition there is a free format report generator which can be used to answer other reporting needs. The ability to batch reports is also present. The report generator is of moderate complexity and can usually be mastered after a little experimentation. Figure 54 shows the main screen.

The general procedure is first to select the patient file from which the search is to be made (more than one file can be included using AND and OR). The selection is then made using drop-down lists from which to choose the exact form of the selection (=, >, etc). The data items to be included in the output can then be selected, as can the order in which they are to appear. There are several different tables all containing a large number of field names and it can be difficult to decide exactly which fields are needed. This approach of exposing the user to the raw data makes quite sophisticated searches possible, but requires the user to refer to the manual to find the fieldname of the required field(s).

Other Systems

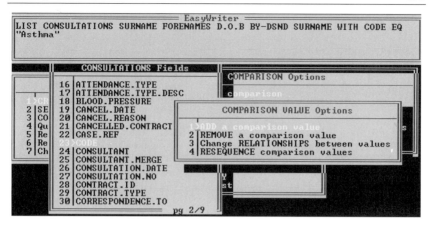

Figure 54 The Amsys report generator

Conclusions

Amsys is a system which is difficult to sum up fairly. This is because aspects of the system that some users might see as advantages might be disadvantages to others. On the one hand, the system is relatively easy to use and contains an easy-to-use Read-code browser and drug dictionary. The report generator is also quite powerful once it has been mastered. On the other hand, the ability to suppress the Read-coded diagnosis, and, more importantly, the drug dictionary, seem to be less impressive as does the rather large number of places where a particular item of information might be stored. It must also be said that from the author's experience of Amsys users they are rather less complimentary about the support offered than is the case with other systems.

At a glance: Amsys

Strengths	Features	Ratings (on a scale of 1–10)
Easy to use with reasonable Read-code implementation. All the basic functions are present. User-defined clinics feature is useful.	Administration/ registration data	✔✔✔
	Consultation data	✔✔
	Reporting	✔✔✔✔
	Templates	✔✔✔
	Integration	✔✔
	Look and feel	✔✔✔
	Costs	✔✔✔
	Support	✔
	Overall	✔✔✔

Weaknesses

Multiple areas for storage of clinical data can cause problems as can the ease with which coded data can be replaced with free text.
    Report generator is initially quite difficult to use.
    Generally unsophisticated.

Seetec GP Professional

Seetec is another popular MS-DOS-based system which is in use in about 300 practices, mostly in the south of England.

Although a hybrid program, Seetec is normally set up to run from Windows 95. The System uses a Local Area Network (LAN), using Windows NT (or occasionally Windows 95) as the networking system.

The system is menu driven and extensive use of function keys is made (these are consistent throughout the program). A mouse can be used to some extent, if desired. The program is written in Clipper (a DBMS system of a type known generically known as 'Xbase'. The main menu screen, with the patients menu dropped down, is shown in Figure 55.

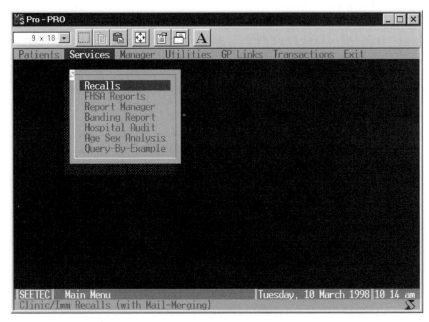

Figure 55   The Seetec GP Professional main menu

Registration Data

As is the case with many of these systems, the registration screen is entirely conventional in use. Again, many of the choices are made from picklists, but in the case of Seetec these are mostly user configurable *at the point of data entry*. If a required choice is not present, simply drop down the picklist, go to the bottom and press the space bar to add the new item. This is rapid and works well in practice, although there is a danger that the same item can be added in two similar but different ways, e.g. SIR and Sir, etc. It is in this way that the address dictionaries can be built up, giving a semi-automatic way of adding address data.

Patient Data

The main methods of entering clinical data into the Seetec system are:

- Consultations
- Non-user definable templates (clinics)

The consultation system can be used either as a problem-based or chronological-based record. Basic consultation details can be added such as date seen, doctor seen, problem description, location (which can be chosen via a picklist) and episode type for the problem-based mode. Multiple entries to the consultation can then be made to categories covering interventions, characteristics and treatments.

The Read-code browser allows selection of the term by rubric and it is relatively easy to move through the Read hierarchy. It is also possible to select a term by its alpha-numeric code. The consultation screen is shown in Figure 56.

The Read-code browser also includes a Read-code formulary allowing the user to filter out codes which are not used. Advanced features include attaching graphical images and sound files to the consultation record. Pathology results received electronically are fully integrated. The QuickCons facility allows the user to enter Read-coded information into the consultation via a practice-defined set of worded abbreviations. A consultation can be moved to either generate a new problem or moved into an existing problem.

As well as the screen discussed above, Seetec contains several specialist screens for chronic disease recording and basic health data. Currently these screens are not user-definable. Figure 57 shows the asthma screen.

134   *Essential Primary Care Computing: A Practice Guide*

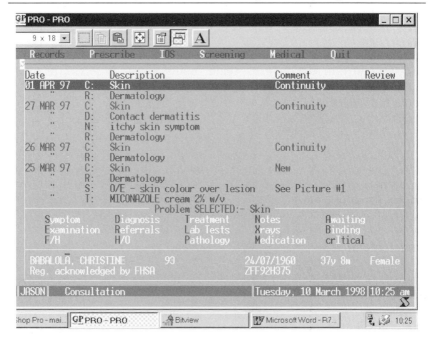

Figure 56   Consultations in Seetec GP Professional

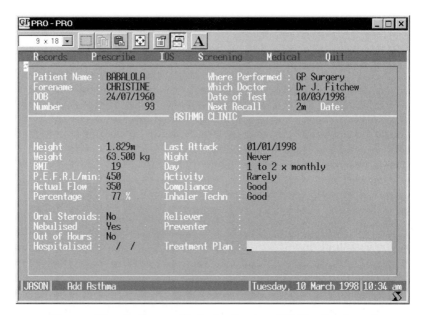

Figure 57   Asthma clinic in Seetec GP Professional

As well as Read coded data and free text, Seetec has a further way of entering coded data by using markers. These are user-defined codes and suffer from the disadvantages mentioned in Chapter 2. Users of the Seetec system still use this facility to some extent, particularly where they feel a Read term does not cover exactly what they want to record.

Prescribing in Seetec GP Professional is straightforward. The drug dictionary used is supplied by Multilex. Sensitivities to drugs and ingredients can be explicitly recorded and there is provision to warn of interactions, drug doubling, precautions, warnings and contra-indications, which are all linked to the consultation system via Read codes. Drugs can be selected from the picking list in the normal way by typing part of their name, or, alternatively, using the product order code, BNF drug chapter, non-drug chapters, user-defined formulary or alternatives such as equivalents, by use or by ingredient. Generic prescribing is also supported. QuickScripts enables the user to set up commonly used practice scripts and to add them quickly to the patient record. The Compliance system shows the frequency that items are prescribed, and a patient's prescription record can be reviewed completely or by individual item.

Referrals are recorded on a specific screen which is linked to the consultation system. Referral letters containing clinical data can be produced semi-automatically using Microsoft Word.

Searches

Standard targets and recalls are performed by predefined reports meeting most of the practices' daily requirements. Custom searches can be designed through the Report Manager which is entirely new in the latest version (Figure 58).

Searches can be grouped in any order and the data exported for use in packages such as Word and Excel, which are supplied with the system.

Conclusions

Seetec, like some of its competitors, is a perfectly adequate clinical computer system for those practices that have moderate needs in relation to clinical data entry. It lacks the sophistication of the major new Windows-based systems, but continues to develop positively. The lack of the single point of storage for a particular item of data in version 2 has now been rectified, but many of the users are happy with it. Seetec users report themselves generally happy with the way their that requests for help are met. The new Version 3 is a significant improvement in terms of both function and stability.

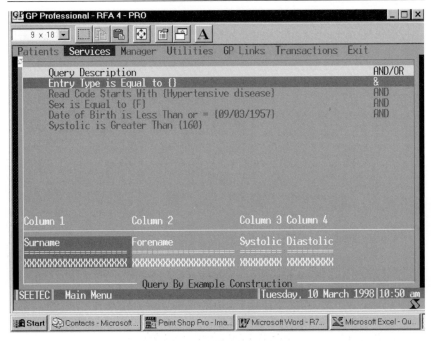

Figure 58 Seetec GP Professional report generator

At a glance: Seetec GP Professional

Strengths	Features	Ratings (on a scale of 1–10)
Competent system which is good value for money, but is easy to use and developing all the time.	Administration/ registration data	✓✓✓✓✓
	Consultation data	✓✓✓✓✓
	Reporting	✓✓✓✓✓
Users report good support from the supplier.	Templates	✓✓
	Integration	✓✓✓
Effective report generator now significantly enhanced.	Look and feel	✓✓✓✓✓
	Costs	✓✓✓✓✓✓✓
	Support	✓✓✓✓✓✓✓
	Overall	✓✓✓✓✓

Weaknesses

Some problems of instability recorded by users, but the situation has improved recently with version 3.0.

Needs user-definable templating system.

Not ideal for paperless use.

Closing Summary

This chapter has sought to describe both the new Windows-based systems from Vamp and AAH Meditel as well as to look brief at a selection of systems from the next tier of suppliers. Clearly, practices hoping to acquire a system should look at as many systems as possible – not just the ones mentioned here. Although the appearance and detailed functionality of the smaller systems vary widely, all are capable of supplying the needs of smaller practices or those who need to input only small amounts of general practice data.

9
Communications

Opening Summary

This chapter summarises the current links used in primary care, namely registration, IOS and pathology. It discusses Email and the uses of the Internet in searching for information. It concludes by discussing briefly how practice systems can be accessed remotely.

Introduction

Communication technology, both within the NHS and in the wider world, is very topical at the moment. Most practices now have registration links directly with their HAs and many have items of service links. A significant number of these practices are also able to receive pathology data directly from the local laboratory.

In addition to this, the Internet is continuing to grow in size at an exponential rate, with both the technology, and the uses to which that technology is put, maturing rapidly.

It would be appropriate first to consider the impact that communications are having on clinical systems.

Registration Links

This first great revolution in the use of clinical systems is now approaching completion, with more than 80% of practices now able to communicate changes in patient registration directly to the HA by using an electronic data link.

Briefly this link, once established, does away with all the time-consuming transmission of paper forms that were once such a major part of the process of registering, de-registering and transferring/ amending the registration of patients. For suitably equipped practices changes and additions are now simply transmitted directly from the general practice system to the HA, where they are picked up directly by the health authority's computer system. As with any new system, there are advantages and disadvantages, but this is one case where the benefits to the NHS as a whole far outweigh the disadvantages. The situation is summarised below:

Advantages:

- Less filling of paper forms
- Accurate practice lists
- Huge efficiency savings at the HA
- Some efficiency savings at the practice

Disadvantages:

- Takes longer to register a patient on the computer than previously
- Certain information must be provided in order to register – cannot be circumvented
- Restrictions on when new patients can be added. Many health authorities do not allow the adding of a new patient during the last week of the quarter

As most practices are now linked for registrations, the debate as to whether a practice should or should not become linked has largely disappeared. In the early stages of this process it is certainly true that many practices experienced teething problems as the software went through the various development stages, and was subsequently refined. Most systems now seem to work reliably and the case for staying out seems weak.

Items of Service Links

The development of links for items of service is one that has a major impact on primary care, making it possible to eliminate most of the paper documentation formerly used for this process. Using the computer for IOS claims also means that mistakes are reduced, as initially the program tends to prompt for the correct information and to ensure that the information entered is consistent.

On most systems the use of IOS links also makes it possible for GPs to complete most of the process from their own consulting rooms merely by entering a few extra details when they enter the claimable Read codes into the system. This means that considerable timesavings can be achieved overall. In addition, delays in payment owing to queries are reduced.

It is difficult to come up with convincing reasons why practices should not adopt IOS links when these are available from their supplier. Clearly, as in any new system, the ongoing costs and the disruption caused by the changeover need to be taken into account, but on the whole the IOS links system is such that it should be in the interests of most practices to become involved.

Although the claims are designed to originate at the point of service, a significant number of practices leave the whole process to a member of the practice staff to administer – particularly in those practices where the GPs seldom use computers. Doing IOS claims in this way seems to work satisfactorily.

Pathology Links

Both the previous types of links are now well established and it is not necessary to deal with them further. Owing to the rather lower take-up of pathology links, we will cover this topic in more detail.

Pathology links allow the transfer of laboratory results (and occasionally requests) to take place electronically between the surgery and the laboratory. In order to illustrate the process, pathology links, as they exist within the EMIS system, are briefly described in the following sections.

Pathology Links – A Practical Example

Pathology links can be used in the areas of haematology, biochemistry, microbiology, histology and cytology, but most laboratories will often only offer a service in some of these areas. Microbiology links often consist of large amounts of free text, which can cause problems of data management. Overall, laboratory links represent a significant saving in time over entering the results manually.

Results received are first held in a 'holding file' where they can be listed or filtered in various ways, e.g. by GP or abnormal only, etc. Figure 59 shows this screen for the EMIS system (*names have been hidden for confidentiality*).

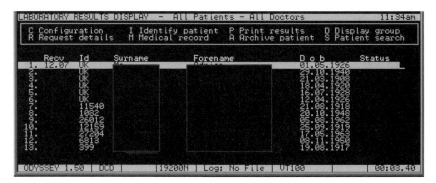

Figure 59   Pathology results in holding file

After a particular result has been highlighted it can be inspected (i.e. the numerical/detail results can be viewed). Figure 60 shows a typical result.

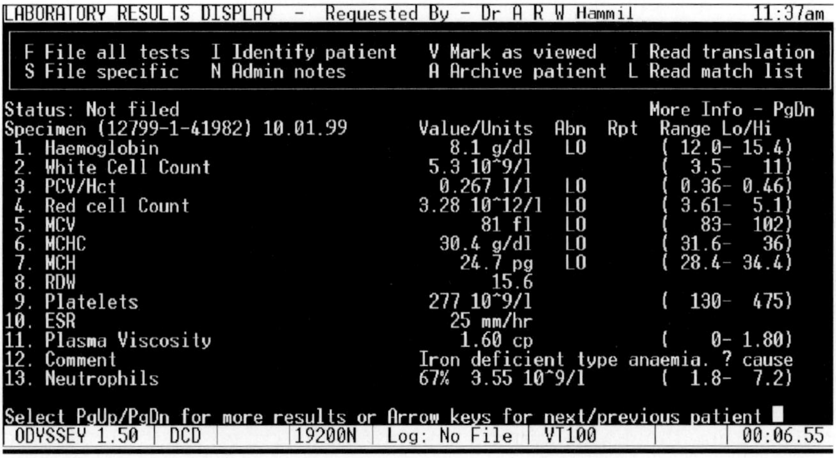

```
LABORATORY RESULTS DISPLAY   -  Requested By - Dr A R W Hammil            11:37am
  F File all tests   I Identify patient    V Mark as viewed    T Read translation
  S File specific    N Admin notes         A Archive patient   L Read match list
Status: Not filed                                              More Info - PgDn
Specimen (12799-1-41982) 10.01.99        Value/Units   Abn  Rpt  Range Lo/Hi
 1. Haemoglobin                             8.1 g/dl    LO       ( 12.0- 15.4)
 2. White Cell Count                        5.3 10^9/1           (  3.5-   11)
 3. PCV/Hct                                 0.267 1/1   LO       ( 0.36- 0.46)
 4. Red cell Count                          3.28 10^12/1 LO      ( 3.61-  5.1)
 5. MCV                                       81 fl     LO       (   83-  102)
 6. MCHC                                    30.4 g/dl   LO       ( 31.6-   36)
 7. MCH                                     24.7 pg     LO       ( 28.4- 34.4)
 8. RDW                                     15.6
 9. Platelets                               277 10^9/1          (  130-  475)
10. ESR                                      25 mm/hr
11. Plasma Viscosity                        1.60 cp            (   0- 1.80)
12. Comment                              Iron deficient type anaemia. ? cause
13. Neutrophils                           67%  3.55 10^9/1      (  1.8-  7.2)
Select PgUp/PgDn for more results or Arrow keys for next/previous patient ■
  ODYSSEY 1.50 | DCD |        |19200N | Log: No File | VT100   |        | 00:06.55
```

Figure 60 Pathology results display

After viewing, results can be transferred to the clinical record, where they appear in the same area as results which have been entered manually. The system can also be set up to transfer 'normal' results from the holding file to the patient record automatically, although opinion is split between GPs as to whether this is a good thing or not.

Other Links

As well as the links mentioned above, many other types of links are envisaged and some of the more likely of these are shown below:

- Email
- Discharge letters
- Death notifications
- Hospital appointments
- Telemedicine

Email

Email is having the ability to send text messages from one computer to another, and to some extent can replace the need to communicate by letter. At its most basic level it allows the exchange of text messages, but most of the software/systems in use allow the *attachment* of files.

This means that a report written, say, in Microsoft Word, can be attached to the Email and sent with it. The recipient can then save the attachment and view/process it in the normal way using the application that created it. Similarly, spreadsheets, databases and other formatted files can also be sent.

There are many different software packages on the market for Email production/receipt, and although they all have there own features, they all do basically the same job.

Most Email provision is via the internet, which allows access worldwide to all other users. Within primary care some individuals are connected via *service providers* in this way, but another option is to connect via the NHS network. This will allow access to other health-care providers in a rather more secure environment than the internet as a whole, as well as providing, in due course, access to the internet via secure gateways. It would seem logical for most primary-care users to connect via the NHS network in due course, although those wishing to connect now may have to use a commercial provider to the internet.

Figure 61 shows an Email message being prepared in the popular Turnpike program. The message is being prepared in an editor, which is really just a very basic word processor.

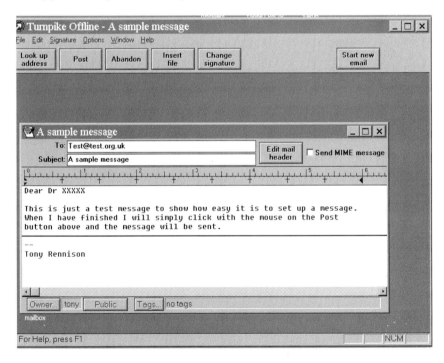

Figure 61   An Email message being prepared

Discharge Letters

Various different types of discharge letter pilots have been carried out. At there simplest level these are simply Email messages that are sent to the practice containing the text of the letter which would normally arrive in paper form. Even at this level of sophistication the system is useful, as the information normally arrives much more quickly at the practice.

At a more sophisticated level, using *EDI* (Electronic Data Interchange) the letter could actually be attached to the patient's record, which would have obvious advantages in terms of access.

Although not possible at the present time, there is no technical reason why a clinical event such as a change of medication actioned in a hospital could not be transmitted directly to the patient's record. When the record is next accessed by the GP, he/she could comply by simply pressing a confirm key.

Most of the above points could also apply to death notifications with the particular benefit that it is always useful for the practice to be aware of deaths as soon as possible.

Hospital Appointments

Although perhaps not currently of such importance in these days of long hospital waiting lists, the ability of a GP to be able to make a hospital appointment for one of his patients from his consulting room, is definitely desirable. Patients would then know immediately where, and more importantly when, they were going to be seen, and the GP would not have to worry so much about patients who have been referred to secondary care, being lost in the system.

The main barriers to this are not technological but more a question of changing attitudes. It is the author's opinion that it will be some time before links such as these are widely available.

Telemedicine

Perhaps one of the ways to reduce hospital outpatient waiting lists is to make greater use of Telemedicine. There are various ways to define Telemedicine, but in essence it allows consultants to consult with patients remotely – normally while the patients are with their GPs.

The system works by having a communications link between the practice and the hospital, with video and sound links via computer systems. The consultant sitting in his office at the hospital can interview the patients and can ask their GPs to carry out various examinations. At its most sophisticated, the GP and the consultant can put on a form of electronic glove which can react if the consultant is examining the patient when the GP is also doing so.

The main problems with Telemedicine are the difficulties in having a sufficiently good link to transmit quality images in real time without huge costs. It is also true to say that some GPs think that the money spent on the link would be better spent on having the consultant hold clinics at the surgery. Even so, this is clearly a developing technology which will allow rural GPs to make better and more efficient use of out-patient services. The cost of providing the hardware to carry out this form of link was, until quite recently, high. With developments in video camera technology and economies of scale, it now costs about £100 to connect a video camera to a PC.

The Internet

It would take several books to describe the internet adequately. In simple terms it is a collection of computer networks linked together that use a common way of communicating with each other. It has its origins in the cold war, when the American defence establishment wanted to build a computer network that could resist direct hits by nuclear weapons on particular sites. Part of its development is also due to the large-scale development of wide-area computer networks in the British university system.

In essence, the World Wide Web (WWW is the name given to this function of the internet) is a method of publishing information and allowing access to all sorts of complex computer databases. Individuals or practices that are equipped with internet access can search the tens of millions of connected sites for relevant information. As well as this, the infrastructure of the internet allows the use of world-wide Email as discussed in an earlier section.

From a medical point of view there are, perhaps, two main uses for the internet:

- To search for information/references to disease and other topics of interest.
- To look at published information (e.g. postgraduate meetings at a centre) which would otherwise only be available on paper.

As examples of the above, if a GP wished to look for information on a disease that he had not encountered previously he could use a *search engine* to search for references to the information. There are many different search engines available on the internet and most work by allowing you to type in keywords, which can then be searched. As an example, Figure 62 show the Alta Vista search engine being used with the Microsoft Internet Explorer browser (a browser is a piece of software that is used to navigate and display information).

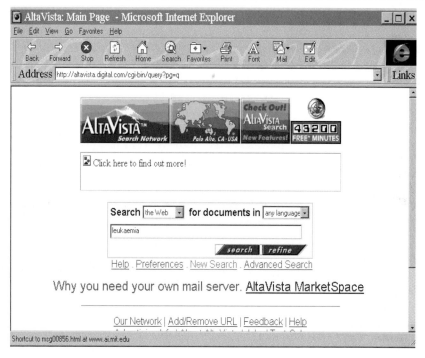

Figure 62 The Alta Vista search engine

Figure 63 shows a few of the results of the search.

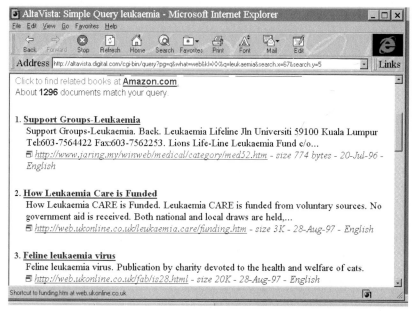

Figure 63 Some results of an internet search

The second use of the internet is to publish information that would only otherwise be available in paper form. Publishing it on the web is more efficient as it saves the distribution costs and can be updated much more easily. Figure 64 is a page taken from the CME+ web site. This is a site that holds details of current educational meetings for GPs throughout the UK.

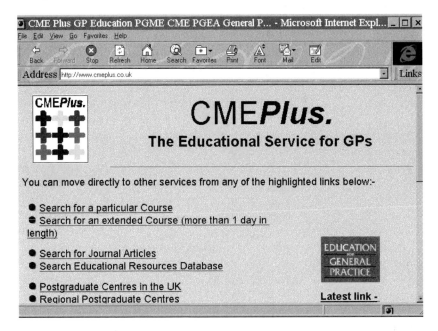

Figure 64 The CME+ web site

All in all the internet is a huge resource which can be of enormous use both to GPs and other members of the practice team. In the next section we will briefly describe the hardware and software that you need to in order to get online.

Hardware and Communications

Hardware and the Internet

In order to get on to the internet you need some way of accessing the connected *backbone* of major computer networks. This is normally achieved by using an internet service provider. This provider – normally a commercial company, but sometimes an academic institution or indeed the NHS – provides you with a means to access the system via a dial-up telephone connection. The hardware/software you need is as follows:

- A normal telephone line – preferably a direct outside line (an ISDN line is even better).
- A PC of adequate speed (the internet, contrary to popular belief, does not need a very powerful PC).
- A modem (or equivalent *terminal adapter* for an ISDN line).
- Suitable communications software.
- An internet browser.

The modem can be internal (i.e. fitted inside the computer case) or external and should be 'fast' enough to make the process of surfing the net bearable. In technical terms this currently means that the modem should be at least 33.6 kb/s in speed, or preferably faster. If you are lucky enough to be able to use an ISDN line, the terminal adapter (i.e. the special modem for ISDN lines) will allow speeds of up to 64 kb/s. If the practice has an existing modem of 14.4 kb/s this can be used, but accessing information will be slower.

Communications software is often supplied by the company providing the link and in any case is built into Windows 95/98 and Windows NT, as is a suitable browser, namely Internet Explorer. An alternative browser, Netscape Navigator, which has similar features, is also available and is preferred by some people.

Setting up the system is much more straightforward than it used to be but in some situations a little skilled technical help may be required. This is often available as a helpline from the service provider. Provided the practice has a suitable PC, to purchase the type of modem required should not cost more than about £100.

Choosing an internet provider can be tricky. All have there strengths and weaknesses, but a major difference between them is the charging structure. Some, including CompuServe and MSN, charge a relatively low monthly fee, but only allow a limited number of hours on-line for this amount. If the time spent on-line exceeds the 'free allowance', it is charged for, and often at quite a high cost. Other suppliers, such as Demon, Pipex, etc charge a higher monthly fee but allow unlimited use, meaning that the only additional cost is the cost of the telephone call.

Most providers have nationwide 'local' numbers so that only local call costs apply, but this is always worth looking into.

Accessing Practice Systems

If a GP or any other member of the practice needs to be able to access the practice system from home, much the same sort of hardware is needed as is needed to connect to the internet. This is a PC, Communications software and a modem. In this case, however, it is likely that a different type of communications software will be needed. Many (but not all) suppliers now support this type of link using standard commercial software. It can be very convenient, for a whole variety of reasons. For GPs, the ability to look up patient records from home, print prescriptions and generally become more proficient at using the system away from the pressures of the practice, are powerful reasons to take advantage of these links, if available.

The whole subject of communications from computer to computer is one which is rapidly expanding. Most practices are now involved in terms of registration and items of service links, and many have access to pathology links and the internet. If you are not currently connected, now is the time to get online and take advantage of these new technologies.

Portable Computers

Increasingly, clinical system suppliers are making use of portable computers in order to allow GPs to access patient records (and in some cases, record data) while away from the practice. In many ways use of such systems is more convenient than a modem link when on the move, as it does not place any reliance on telephone lines or portable telephones.

10
Using PCs in General Practice

Opening Summary

This chapter describes some of the uses that standard PCs have in the practice. Spreadsheets are looked at in some detail. Word processing, accounts, DTP, presentation software and personal information managers are also mentioned. The topic of transferring clinical information to a PC is discussed.

Introduction

Standard business computers – for the purposes of this book those that use MS-DOS/Windows or Windows 95/98 as their operating system – are used in most sections of industry and commerce.

In the past the majority of general practice systems did not use MS-DOS/Windows as their operating system. Because of this and because of the fact that in the past suppliers have made little effort to allow the transfer of clinical data to an MS-DOS/Windows environment, the use of standard business computers in general practice has not advanced as far as it might have done.

It could be said that in some circumstances a stand-alone computer running ordinary business applications can have as much cost/benefit as a clinical system! Although this is true, maximum benefit can only be gained if the transfer of clinical data from the medical system is possible. All the 'new' systems now being produced have at least some facility for the *export* of data to applications such as word processors and spreadsheets.

There are many different types of applications software available for PCs. Some types of software are not relevant to general practice. The following list indicates the main types of application which can be of use:

- Spreadsheets
- Word processing
- Accounts
- Databases – other than main clinical system
- Payroll

Spreadsheets

Spreadsheets can be of major use to a practice and yet many practice staff are not aware of their function. This is unfortunate as spreadsheets (with word processing) are possibly the two most useful pieces of software for the practice to use, after their clinical system. Spreadsheets have two major uses in general practice:

1. Numerical analysis
2. Presentation of data

Numerical analysis, in its simplest sense, is the spreadsheet's ability to recalculate a set of calculations automatically when the data is changed. For example, consider a spreadsheet which has been set up to calculate items of service income as it appears on the HA return, in terms of the number of items in each category and their value. Using the spreadsheet, the total value of each item can be calculated again and again by simply changing the input, in this case the number of, for example, night visits.

The presentation of data is the other major use of spreadsheets, i.e. to present data in graphical form. Spreadsheets make it very easy to produce a wide variety of charts in very little time. It is often the case that the results of medical audit are best presented graphically. Charts produced in spreadsheets can be exported to other packages such as word-processors.

Spreadsheet Development

Spreadsheets have been around for as long as there have been personal computers and they have today developed into very powerful financial and scientific tools. VisiCalc was probably the first viable spreadsheet program for micros. This program, introduced in 1978, was the most popular software product around at the time, selling about half a million copies. In the 1980s, Lotus 123 became the spreadsheet of choice for the majority of users and was the market leader for many years.

Nowadays Microsoft Excel is the clear market leader. An Excel spreadsheet is shown in Figure 65.

Here are definitions of some of the important terms used in spreadsheets:

- *Columns* are the vertical arrangement of *cells*, and are headed A, B, C, etc and then AA, AB, AC, etc ... BA, BB, BC, ...
- *Rows* are the horizontal rows of cells, and are numbered, 1, 2, 3, 4, ... up to at least 9999.

Using PCs in General Practice 153

- *Cells* are the places where rows and columns intersect, and are known by references such as A6 or B4.

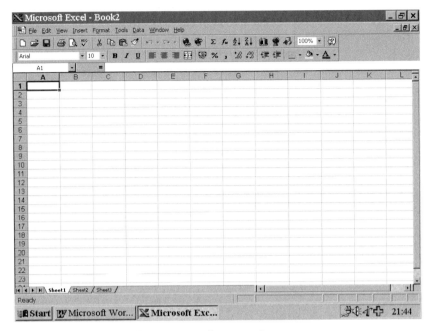

Figure 65 The Excel screen

Modern spreadsheets now generally offer three-dimensional operation, hence in some programs 'tabs' appear with the symbols A, B, C or 1, 2, 3, etc at the bottom of the screen to indicate the constituent pages of the spreadsheet.

Essentially cells can contain three different types or entry:

- Labels
- Data
- Formula

Labels are text entries that are present to show what the numbers in a spreadsheet refer to. They would include entries such as 'Total' and 'Gross Profit', as well as titles such as 'No. of Minor Ops by Category in 1991'.

Data are the numbers which are used in the spreadsheet (or, more properly, worksheet), e.g. 123.81, 6e, –2, 125471.3, which are are all valid data values.

Formula are the entries which manipulate numbers in order to give calculated results, e.g.

- summing a group of cells
- multiplying one cell by another

- adding 1.03 to a cell's contents

Figure 66 is a typical spreadsheet that might be used in General Practice. It is a practice income spreadsheet. All the various sources of income to the practice have been identified and grouped in logical sections, and are displayed in the left-most column of the spreadsheet. Each quarter's actual income can then be entered in the appropriate column. This example can be produced with various levels of sophistication, depending on the requirements and the skill of the user. At the very least, income per patient can be calculated and compared with the national average. At a more sophisticated level, charts showing practice income in various categories can be produced. Figure 67 shows such a chart.

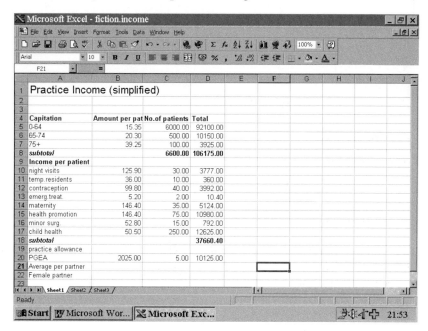

Figure 66   Simple practice income example

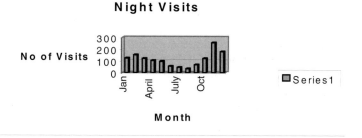

Figure 67   Charting using Excel

Another example of a useful spreadsheet is the electronic cashbook. This is an electronic form of a manual ledger and can be set up in a very short time (less half an hour). It has the same features as an ordinary cashbook but never makes mistakes in the arithmetic. Also, if a value is entered in error, it can easily be corrected and all subsequent balances in the cashbook are automatically amended. Figure 68 shows such a spreadsheet.

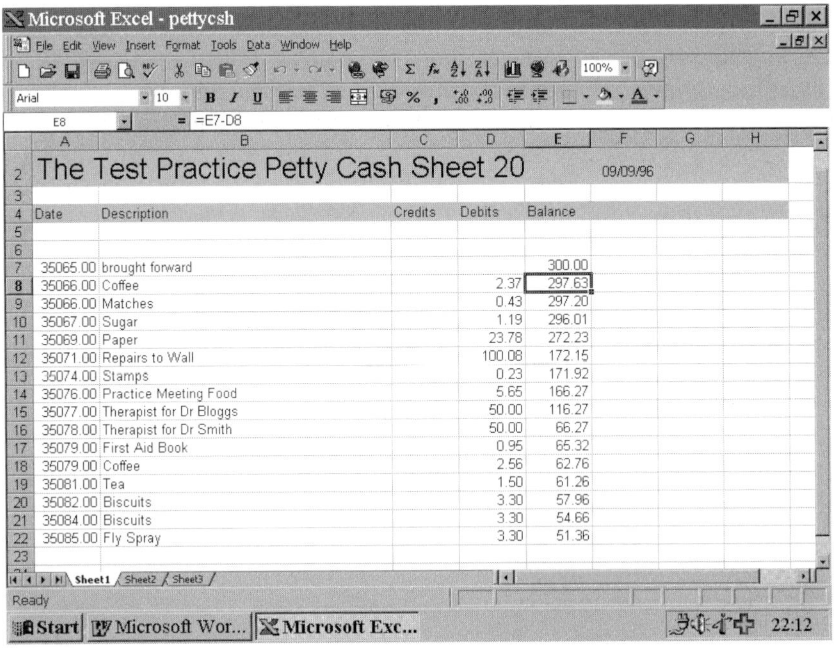

Date	Description	Credits	Debits	Balance
35065.00	brought forward			300.00
35066.00	Coffee		2.37	297.63
35066.00	Matches		0.43	297.20
35067.00	Sugar		1.19	296.01
35069.00	Paper		23.78	272.23
35071.00	Repairs to Wall		100.08	172.15
35074.00	Stamps		0.23	171.92
35076.00	Practice Meeting Food		5.65	166.27
35077.00	Therapist for Dr Bloggs		50.00	116.27
35078.00	Therapist for Dr Smith		50.00	66.27
35079.00	First Aid Book		0.95	65.32
35079.00	Coffee		2.56	62.76
35081.00	Tea		1.50	61.26
35082.00	Biscuits		3.30	57.96
35084.00	Biscuits		3.30	54.66
35085.00	Fly Spray		3.30	51.36

Figure 68 Using Excel as a cashbook

As already mentioned, extracting data from practice systems can be difficult in some cases, but it is in this situation where spreadsheets can be of most use in clinical medicine. If, for example, an audit has been conducted using the clinical system, *provided the facility exists*, the data can be 'downloaded' to a PC and charts can be created with no further data entry. If the clinical system in question does not support the export of data, the charts can still be drawn, but the data will have to be re-entered into the spreadsheet.

To summarise, spreadsheets are a useful tool in general practice information handling. Training in their use is normally available from a variety of sources including local colleges, commercial training providers, CME groups, MAAGS and sometimes HAs. If you have a PC in the practice capable of running a spreadsheet, learning how to use it can be of great benefit.

Word Processing

Word processing (WP) is the most popular application used on PCs. It is also the application that is most widely understood by those persons not otherwise familiar with computer software. Although most people have some knowledge of word processing, many are unaware of the range of features available in modern WP software.

Although most clinical systems have some form of built-in WP facilities, so as to be able to produce standard letters and other documents, the features of these built-in systems do not normally compare with the popular mainstream stand-alone software. Sometimes systems are able to incorporate 'external' WP software and hence to replace the more simplistic provision that was built-in originally. This can be useful, as the range of formatting options for letters is then much greater as well as offering the possibility of much more professional practice reports. Windows programs allow the option of having a number of documents to be 'open' or active at the same time, with the consequent ability to transfer portions of text easily between them. Additionally, programs running under Windows normally display documents identically to how they will finally appear on the printed paper (What You See Is What You Get – WYSIWYG). This can be very helpful.

Often hundreds of fonts (typestyles) are available in a large range of sizes, as well as precise control over virtually every aspect of the layout of documents. Many of the features of the latest software may be of limited use in the day-to-day running of general practice, although items such as automatic envelope printing and comprehensive spell-checking are normally welcomed.

As with spreadsheets, there is a limited number of packages in widespread use and the main titles are very similar in terms of the vast range of features that they offer.

Microsoft Word

Currently the most popular word processor in the world and one which is due to be upgraded and released in 1999 for the latest version of Windows (Windows 98). It can be purchased singly but is often supplied as part of a package called Microsoft Office. This includes Microsoft Excel, the presentation software PowerPoint and an organiser called Outlook.

Corel WordPerfect

WordPerfect used to produce the popular MS-DOS word processor of the same name, but it has had less success with its Windows version.

The features of this package are similar to those of Word, although users of the MS-DOS version of WordPerfect might well prefer it to Word. The program is also available as part of the software suite, Corel Office – this time including the Windows version of the spreadsheet Quattro Pro.

Lotus Word Pro

This is the third of the major word processor packages on the market, and comes from the spreadsheet makers Lotus, now owned by IBM. It again has a wealth of features which make it very similar in functionality to the other two. It is also often supplied as part of Lotus Smartsuite, which contains the Lotus spreadsheet.

Accounts Software

Accounts is an application which many practices wish to implement either as an add-on to their clinical system or as a stand-alone package on a PC. Small practices with relatively simple accounts should consider carefully if the work involved in computerisation is worthwhile in terms of the advantages which computerisation brings.

So what are the advantages and disadvantages of computerised accounting?

Advantages

- System handles all the calculations – no mistakes in the arithmetic.
- Easy access to cost analysis, i.e. How much was spent on heat and light in last 12 months?
- Up-to-date totals for income and expenditure – easy to keep track of the financial situation.

Disadvantages

- Another program to learn.
- Duplicate data entry – a manual system of books should be maintained, at least until the computer system is fully validated.
- Most accounts packages are double entry – can be complicated both to understand and to amend.

Many of the clinical suppliers can supply an accounts package to run on the same hardware as the main system. In some cases these are supplied at no additional cost. There are also a small number of accounts packages written specifically for GPs by other third-party suppliers.

The advantage of systems from the clinical supplier is that they are normally designed to work on the same hardware (and with the same operating systems) as the clinical system. They have also been designed from the outset for use in general practice and so are not encumbered with unnecessary features such as VAT analysis. However, in some cases they are rather expensive and can be rather poorly developed compared with standard accounting packages designed for PCs. Additionally, in a number of cases the on-going charges of these systems can be higher. The specialist third-party software shares most of the advantages mentioned above but, as specialist software, is considered by many GPs to be superior.

As well as the above types of accounts packages, a large number of standard commercial accounts software packages such as Quicken and Money are also available, often at very low cost. The standard of this software can be very high. The main disadvantage is that these systems have been developed for general business use and, as such, tend to have a whole range of complex features which are of little use in general practice. As well as VAT, most of these packages will be based around the concept of monthly figures, whereas owing to the nature of quarterly payments in general practice, this period is more important.

In the final analysis the same basic criteria apply to purchasing accounts software as to clinical software. It is important to have a clear idea of the major objectives and also to look at as many systems as possible. The situation is perhaps a little more complex owing to the number of different types of accounts packages available, as detailed above. In the end the very low cost of major mainstream commercial packages has to be weighed against the more specialist and more expensive software designed for GP use.

Other Software

There is a whole range of additional software that can, in the right circumstances, be useful in the practice. These include:

- Desk-top publishing
- Presentation software
- Personal information managers (PIMs)
- Distance learning material
- Reference material
- Payroll
- Non-clinical database systems

Desk-top Publishing

Desk-top publishing software gives the practice the ability to produce leaflets and 'printed' forms, brochures and newsletters. A few years ago not only was the software expensive and complex, but also adequate hardware was costly.

This has now all changed and adequate easy-to-use software can be obtained for less than £100. Although the heavyweight packages such as CorelDraw, Ventura Publisher and Aldus PageMaker are still available, practices would normally be well advised to consider packages like Serif PagePlus or Microsoft Publisher, which will satisfy most normal requirements.

In a significant number of cases even a good word processor will fulfil a lot of what a DTP package can do, although it may take a little longer to produce equivalent results.

If embarking on DTP work, it is important to make sure that a good-quality printer is available. A reasonable laser printer is probably the best option, although an inkjet can produce good results and is the only practical option if colour work is envisaged.

Presentation Software

Often GPs and other practice staff are involved in the educational process and presentation software can be very useful to produce overhead transparencies and handouts.

Whereas effective overhead transparencies and slides can be produced with an ordinary word processor, the result is normally much more professional if a presentation package is used. It is also easier and quicker. Microsoft, as part of the 'Office' package, supplies PowerPoint. Another well known packages is Harvard Graphics.

Personal Information Managers (PIMs)

PIMs (or electronic diaries) are available in a variety of forms – from those that run on the tiny Psion Organiser to programs for PCs. All have their place, but we will first consider those which are used on PCs.

These programs can be very useful if they are well managed and can make the process of maintaining a practice diary so much easier. Both the form and the layout of these programs vary widely, but all allow entries to be entered against times/dates with a wide range of output options. They all also normally allow repetitive entries to be entered automatically so that, for example, if the practice always has a meeting at 1200 on a Wednesday, this can then appear automatically. Most offer alarms and the ability to maintain multiple diaries.

Electronic organisers range in price from about £40 to about £500, depending on the features that they offer. At the bottom end of the price range, they are basically glorified calculators with some diary (and sometimes note-taking) ability. Data is not normally transferable by electronic means to a PC. At the top end, comprehensive diary management is offered along with word processing and spreadsheet ability. The ability to share data with a PIM running on a PC is often also supported.

If many people need to share diary information then some form of PIM running on a PC can be a very good idea. It does take a certain commitment to adjust to a different way of working, but allows a master diary to be maintained easily. It is then possible to print in Filofax format so that individuals can carry a paper version around with them. Problems can arise, however, if individuals make appointments and then fail to enter these on to the program!

Distance Learning Material

Another use for PCs is distance learning packages. Many of these packages now exist and are a useful way of refreshing knowledge in a particular area of medicine. The main advantages over text-based systems are threefold:

- Individuals can work at their own pace at times convenient to them.
- Computer-based learning can be much more interactive than is the case with book-based learning.
- In the most recent software (and given a suitably equipped PC), video and sound can be used to produce a multimedia environment.

Computer-based assessment is now available in a variety of subject areas, and assessment, combined with suitably targeted educational material, makes for a very powerful educational medium.

Reference Material

Various on-line sources of information are now available to GPs who have access to a PC equipped with some communications software and a modem. Typical of these is Medline, run by the BMA, which allows on-line access to medical abstracts which can be searched in a variety of ways, and BioMedNet which is a web site for health professionals and those working in related fields.

Various medical bulletin boards also exist which allow GPs to discuss with others their views and opinions in an on-line environment.

Payroll

Traditionally payroll has either been calculated manually using tables supplied by the Inland Revenue or else a spreadsheet has been constructed to take care of the calculations. All this is now redundant as effective stand-alone payroll programs are available for very little outlay. These programs, which are normally kept up-to-date with changes in the tax system by means of update disks, make the whole process of calculating tax and National Insurance contributions very simple.

Non-clinical Database Systems

A whole range of commercial DBMSs (database management systems) are available including Access (part of Microsoft Office, Professional Edition) and Paradox by Borland. These systems enable practices to set up simple databases for themselves and can be useful in the situation where the clinical system is unable to carry out the required task. Although less likely to be needed with more modern clinical software, it must still be borne in mind that in many cases existing data from the clinical system will have to be re-entered by hand. You should only use these systems if you have a clearly defined need that can be met in no other way.

Integration with the Clinical System

Much of the software that has been mentioned in this chapter is much more useful if it can be integrated with data from the clinical system. This means that data can be sent directly from the clinical system to the software application in question. Examples are sending clinical data to a spreadsheet for further processing, or a list of names and addresses to a word processor for mail merging. Note that the flow of information is only in one direction. It is not generally possible or desirable at the current stage of development to send information in the other direction.

If the system is using a non-MS-DOS/Windows operating system, the situation is sometimes more complicated, but in simple terms it is necessary for the clinical system to have some method of creating an MS-DOS/Windows-type file on a disk. The *format* of the file is normally ASCII. ASCII is a standard way of creating text files which contain no special formatting information and it has become a standard method of transferring information between computers. A particular form of ASCII file that is very popular for transferring data records from one system to another is the delimited file, most commonly the comma-delimited file.

In a delimited file no special formatting is present (ASCII text) and each *record* exists on its own line separated from other records by a hard return. Each *field* is separated or *delimited* from other fields by some other character, usually a comma. Other common file formats are Excel .XLS or Lotus .WK? spreadsheet formats, and dBase datafile format .DBF.

Some clinical systems do not have any easy way of exporting data to an MS-DOS/Windows-type file in ASCII format. In these cases other more complex methods of exporting the data have to be employed. Generally this involves trying to copy printer spooler files to MS-DOS or even to re-direct the printed output to an MS-DOS file by replacing the printer with a PC. Such methods should only be attempted by those who know exactly what they are doing.

In order to show the principles of using a clinical system with a standard WP system, the task of transferring information from an AAH Meditel System 5 clinical system and an EMIS system to Word is considered next.

AAH Meditel uses the Lyrix WP program which is well integrated into the clinical system. This WP package, although quite satisfactory for the majority of standard tasks, does not compare favourably to a more modern Windows-based WP system. It might well be the case that a report generated in the AAH Meditel system would then be moved to Word in order to tidy it up and generally improve its appearance.

To achieve this after saving the report in the AAH Meditel system it is necessary to exit the AAH Meditel system and go to the XENIX command prompt. Providing the exact location of the document in the XENIX directory structure is known, the document can be exported to an MS-DOS/Windows-formatted floppy disk. This can be done using the XENIX command DOSCP followed by the path to the document and either X: or Y: depending on the type of floppy drive on the AAH Meditel machine. If the filename is longer than the eight characters allowed by the MS-DOS file system, it will be truncated.

Having copied the file on disk, it can then be transferred to a machine running Word and imported as shown in Figure 69. It is likely that some formatting information, such as lines, may have to be removed as they may not appear correctly. The document can then be formatted as desired before printing.

To use EMIS to achieve the same result, first produce a search in the normal way. Then, using 'search results', select 'save to an ASCII file'. Fields for inclusion in the MS-DOS output file can then be selected. Finally the file is written to a floppy disk in the file server. This file can then be loaded into Word, as in the case of AAH Meditel, as before.

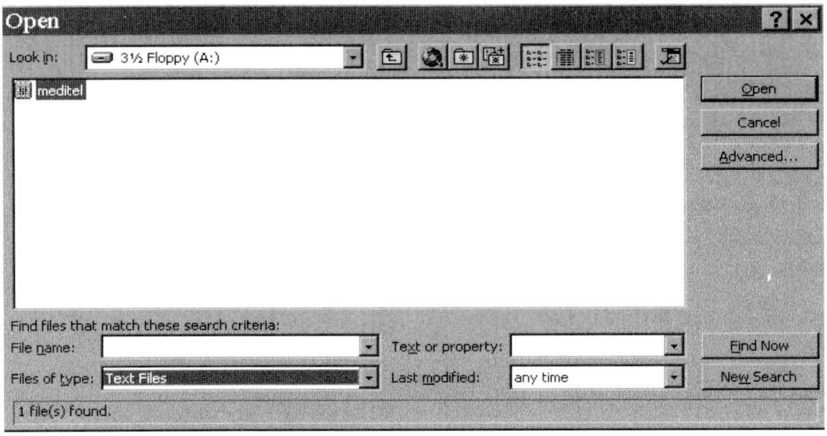

Figure 69 Opening a text file in Word

Closing Summary

The use of PCs in general practice is one that could fill many books, and this chapter is little more than an introduction to some of the software which may be useful.

Without doubt, the most useful non-clinical software for most practices is a good word processing package, and perhaps also a spreadsheet. It has been said that, for many practices, acquiring these two items is probably far more cost-effective than the best-value clinical system on the market.

Appendix 1
Glossary of Terms

The following is not meant to be an exhaustive glossary of terms, but rather a brief explanation of some of the terms mentioned in the text.

Bus In simple terms, the connecting paths connecting all the main components of the system together.

Byte A quantity of information loosely equivalent to one character.

CPU/Processor The calculating part of the computer that actually carries out the processing in programs.

Disk/Diskette Permanent storage. **Diskette** refers to floppy drives whereas **disk** is interchangeable.

EISA A now obsolete enhanced version of the **ISA** bus.

Field The place where a particular item of information from a **Record** is stored. For example, in a patient registration table each record would have a field for the surname.

GUI (Graphical User Interface) A Windows-type system, as distinct from a text-based (often terminal-based) one.

ISA Traditionally the most common type of expansion slot to find in a computer for adding extra hardware such as sound cards, internal modems, etc. Still often found but now being superseded by **PCI**.

LAN (Local Area Network) A method of connecting a number of computers together that has some distinct advantages over a multi-user set-up.

Listmatching The process of reconciling the Heath Authorities' patient registration with the information on the same patients held by the practice.

Macro A recorded series of keystrokes enabling a complex operation to be carried out easily by *playing* the macro back. For example, in Vamp Medical, there are many keystrokes needed to add a history entry for cystitis, add a prescription for trimethoprim and print it, but the whole process can be recorded as a macro and actioned using three key presses.

Modem A device to allow computers to pass data down ordinary telephone lines. Used to connect to the internet and for links.

Mouse A small electro-mechanical pointing device moved by the hand with two or three buttons on it. Used in a **GUI** operating system to carry out operations such as opening menus and confirming actions.

Multiplexor A device that allows a large number of serial ports to be attached to one central computer.

Multi-user system A system based on one central computer and a number of terminals (or PCs running terminal-emulation software).

MUMPS The operating system used by EMIS and the Exeter general practice system. Runs on top of MS-DOS.

OXMIS A medical term-coding system used in Vamp Medical and a few others. Now superseded by Read.

PC Personal computer – an IBM-compatible machine as distinct to an Apple Macintosh or an Archimedes.

PCI The latest type of expansion card slot. Superior to ISA/EISA.

RAM (Random Access Memory) The memory in a computer that is available to run programs and store data. It can be considered to be the computer's 'thinking space'. Also see **ROM**. The quantity of RAM is measured in megabytes (Mb) and is normally at least 16 Mb in a PC.

Record A set of **Fields**, i.e. in a patient registration table, all the information for John Smith.

ROM (Read Only Memory) A type of memory that contains information which cannot be altered. Normally used to supply the computer with basic instructions on how to load the operating system, but also has other uses.

Rubric A test term that describes a Read code (or more generally any other type of code), e.g. asthma is the rubric for H33.

Run-time A system that can be run but not modified (as in SOPHIE).

RSI (Repetitive Strain Injury) Caused by spending too much time with limbs in certain fixed positions when using a computer. The subject of some controversy.

Server The central machine in a network that shares its files and sometimes other resources such as modems.

Sound card An add-on card that allows sound to be produced by the computer.

Terminal A dumb screen and keyboard used by multi-user-based systems.

Terminal Emulation A method of making a PC behave as if it is a terminal using software.

UPS (Uninterruptible Power Supply) A unit placed between the mains power source and a computer (normally the server) to prevent disruption and problems due to supply failure. The unit senses the mains voltage and activates if it drops below a certain level, using internal batteries to maintain power to the system.

Virus *See* Appendix 4

Appendix 2
Recommended *Minimum* Specification for a Server

Bear in mind that this is the minimum recommended specification for a server Always go for the best specification that is appropriate as it is often more expensive to upgrade later

- Tower-type floor-standing case
- Pentium II processor running at a minimum of 300 MHz
- 128 Mb of RAM
- 6 Gb hard disk, ideally mirrored (or else a RAID array)
- Adequate tape back-up system, preferably DAT capable of backing up the whole system to one tape
- The video card specification and monitor are relatively unimportant on a server unless it is to have a workstation role as well.

Appendix 3
Recommended *Minimum* Specification for a PC Workstation

Bear in mind that this is the minimum recommended specification for a workstation Always go for the best specification that is appropriate as it is often more expensive to upgrade later

- Tower or desktop case, as appropriate
- Pentium P233 MMX processor
- 32 Mb RAM
- 3 Gb hard disk
- 512 kb secondary cache
- 2 Mb RAM video card
- 15 inch monitor (XGA)
- Windows 95/98 or NT 4.0
- Microsoft Office
- 2 serial ports (high speed)

Appendix 4
The Essentials of Virus Protection

What is a PC Virus?

A virus is a small malevolent program that attaches itself to part of your system and can very easily spread throughout your PC. It is introduced to the system by infected files normally originating from a floppy disk or the internet. While acknowledging that some of the viruses will create immense damage to your data, even the less harmful and innocuous viruses should be eliminated as they waste disk space, time and may accidentally corrupt data. They are normally written by computer 'nerds' with very serious personality disorders who find it amusing to waste everybody else's time.

Types of Viruses

New types of viruses are emerging all the time, but the following are the broad categories into which they can be classified.

Boot/Partition Sector Virus

These are often spread by the use of infected floppy disks, including accidentally allowing the system to boot up when the infected floppy is in the drive. If a message such as 'Not a system disk ...' is displayed, it may be too late as your hard disk may already have been infected! Because the boot sector of the disk is involved, these viruses are often harder to remove than others. Also, because these viruses then enter the system via the boot sector of the hard disk of the machine, it is difficult to remove them from RAM. It is also very easy to contaminate 'emergency boot disks' with this type of virus.

'Normal' Viruses

These are small programs that attach themselves to existing files with .COM and .EXE extensions, i.e. to program files. They often originate in dubious games software on floppy disk or in downloadable 'free' software available on the internet. When the infected program is started, the virus code installs itself in RAM and then allows the program to run normally. The virus code then attaches itself to other program files that are run. It can also start to corrupt files and to do whatever damage it has been programmed to carry out. This can range from harmless messages displayed at certain times to rendering the entire hard disk useless until it is reformatted, with the consequent total loss of all information held on it. At this point it should be emphasised that viruses cannot harm the hardware of your machine under normal circumstances. However, it is possible theoretically for a virus to be written that could physically damage a monitor or a BIOS, but thankfully so far these have not appeared – yet.

Windows-specific Viruses

These are viruses that specifically exploit the Windows operating system by making use of a feature something called the API so as to inflict damage. They are relatively rare but are often very harmful, as they disable or change the normal action of menu commands. For example, they can disable the File Save function without telling you.

Macro Viruses

The code for these viruses is actually in a macro language which is used by word processing and spreadsheet programs. Usually the viruses infect a template, so that future documents created or used that are based on that template will be infected. Most of them infect Microsoft Word, partly because Word documents are often attached to Emails and partly because a significant number of people use this program as their Email editor.

Types of Anti-virus Software

It is possible to protect your PC from further invasion and also to track down and eliminate existing viruses. Many anti-virus software packages are now available, and most are made up of program elements for scanning and monitoring.

Scanners

Scanners normally work by scanning hard disks and floppy disks for the 'signatures' (i.e. the unique program code) of known viruses. When a virus is encountered, the software will, in most cases, be able to 'disinfect' it, thus neutralising the threat. Scanners work in many different ways and are evolving into very sophisticated tools as the viruses themselves become more and more aggressive.

Monitors

Monitors are programs that observe system activity and can note changes being made to the master boot record of the primary hard disk and/or any other unusual signs. They work by prevention, identifying the problem immediately, rather than repairing problems discovered in a scan. Monitors can also be used to monitor incoming Email and other internet traffic that might be dangerous; some can be programmed to enforce security on a system by, for example, disallowing the downloading of 'cookies' – small, often legitimate, programs downloaded to your machine via your web-browsing software for a variety of purposes by (in the main) software suppliers.

There is also software available that can be used to enforce a degree of physical security on a PC or a group of networked PCs. These systems make it impossible for floppies to be read by the PCs in the group, thus preventing the introduction of viruses. Obviously, the implementation of this software must be done on machines that are known to be 'clean' initially.

Prevention – the Adoption of Rules and Procedures

It is necessary to adopt and to follow a few basic rules and procedures in order to prevent the inconvenience caused by viruses attacking your system:

1. Regularly use your anti-virus software to scan your hard disk. From time to time, scan the whole system from the emergency floppy boot disk which is normally created as part of the anti-virus software installation.
2. Never leave a floppy disk in a floppy drive when you turn off/turn on the PC.
3. If someone has used their own floppy disks on your PC, scan your hard disk immediately.
4. Never use pirated software or illegal copies of programs or games.
5. Be very reluctant to use floppy disks in your machine originating from other people. If this is unavoidable, make sure that they have used effective virus protection and, in any event, always scan any floppy disks immediately.
6. The internet is currently the source of many of the viruses that

affect people. Apart from having effective anti-virus software, it is sensible to transfer files in a form that cannot be infected with viruses. In relation to word processed material, this probably means using an alternative format such as RTF (rich text format) rather than Microsoft Word format. Although less convenient, spreadsheets are probably better sent and received as textual ASCII files.
7. Make sure that you subscribe to the regular updates that are available for your virus software so that it will have a better chance of recognising the latest viruses.

Above all, do not be too worried. Although viruses are now common, the really nasty ones are still relatively rare. However, virus infection is something that can definitely happen to you, so equip yourself with one of the leading anti-virus packages if you do not already have one, and think carefully about the possibility of virus infection via floppy disk or the internet.

Suggested Anti-virus Software

The following packages should give reasonable protection if used carefully and as suggested by their suppliers:

1. *Dr Solomon's Anti-Virus Toolkit* – Dr Solomon's Software
2. *McAfee VirusScan* – Network Associates
3. *Norton AntiVirus* – Symantec

Appendix 5
Suppliers Mentioned in the Text

System	Supplier
Vamp Medical	Reuters Health Information Ltd, Smugglers Way, London SW18 1EG; ☎ 0171–498 1330
Vamp Vision	As above
System 5	AAH Meditel Ltd, Rigby Hall, Rigby Lane, Bromsgrove, Worcs B60 2EW; ☎ 01527–579414
System 6000	As above
EMIS	Egton Medical Information Systems Ltd, Park House Mews, 77 Back Lane, off Broadway, Horsforth, Leeds LS18 4RF; ☎ 0113–259 1122
Amsys	LK Global Healthvare Systems (UK) Ltd, Theobald Business Centre, Knowle Piece, Wilbury Way, Hitchin, Herts SG4 0TY; ☎ 01462–755100
Ambridge	Torex Medical Ltd, 3 Blenheim Court, Lustleigh Close, Matford, Exeter EX2 8PW; ☎ 01392–203522
GP Professional	Seetec Medical Systems, Main Road, Hockley, Essex SS5 4RG; ☎ 01702–201070

In addition to the above, there are many other GP systems suppliers. Lists of suppliers appear in *Practice Computing* magazine and *Medeconomics*. Other systems with significant numbers of users include:

Supplier	System	Contact	Phone number
Chime	Paradoc	GP Care	0171–288 5209
Brandt Computer Systems Ltd	Medico		01293–771361
Exeter GP Systems	Exeter System		01257–262539
HollowBrook Computer Services	Micro-Doc		0114–268 4582
M-Tech Computer Services	HMC		01603–870620

At the time of writing, a number of companies were in merger talks, check the sources quoted above for the most up-to-date information.

Appendix 6
Further Reading

It is difficult to recommend books specifically on general practice computing as there are only a few of these – unlike books on practice accounting, etc of which there are many. However, the following list may be of use:

1. *The Use of Computers in General Practice*, John Preece, Churchill Livingstone (1994. Deals in a rigorous way with many of the principles involved in practice computing, and is recommended.
2. *Making Sense of Computers in General Practice*, Allen and Quinlan, Radcliffe (1995). Does not deal with specific systems but contains a lot of useful information about the business/administration side of practice computing. The *Making Sense of* series contains a number of titles.
3. *Practice Information Management and Technology*, Information Management Group, NHS (1995). A mixture of disk- and text-based aids that can be used to show the role of IT in primary care.

There are many books on spreadsheets, databases, word processors and the internet, and readers need to find those which refer to the specific software they use. Often computer books are quite expensive and care needs to be taken over their selection. Of particular note, however, are:

1. *10 Minute Guides*, various authors, Que. Excellent if you wish to become proficient quickly in using a particular program.
2. *Dummies Guides*, various authors, IDG Books. Again a valuable series of books on most popular software programs, with a no-nonsense style.
3. *Running Microsoft Office 97*, Halvorson and Young, Microsoft Press (1997). Microsoft are in a good position to publish books on their products (although perhaps they ought to call them manuals and include them when you buy the software!), and this is the latest in a series of good general introductions to the use of this package. Microsoft also produce good, if weighty, volumes on Windows 95 and Windows NT.

Generally, if you are going to buy a book or books on computing it is

Appendix 6: Further Reading

worth seeking out your nearest large bookshop (Dillons, Waterstones, etc) and allow yourself plenty of time to make your selection. There is nothing worse than spending £40–£50 on a book only to find that, apart from a pretty cover, it has little to recommend it over the manuals supplied with the software that you have purchased.

Index

80286 15
80386 15
80486 15
8088/8086 14

A4 records 2
AAH Meditel 7, 11, 27, 60, 62, 64, 67–81, 86, 88–89, 92, 98, 107, 113–120, 122, 123, 127, 129, 137, 162, 173
Abnormal values 63
Age–sex registers 8, 22
AGP 14
ANA 76
Annual reports 5, 64
Appointment systems 5, 35, 79, 127
Arbitrary (code) 26
Arnet multiplexers 81
ASCII 9, 79, 91, 112, 118, 161, 162, 172
AT 13
ATX 13
Audit 3–5, 10, 11, 23, 58, 59, 63, 64, 89, 91, 152, 155
Audit trail 23
Automatic reordering 31

Back Office system 21
Backups 2, 58, 59
Basic health data 10, 21, 49, 59, 104, 133
BOS 18, 95
British Computer Society 34
Cache 14, 16, 168
Capital costs 8, 22, 23
Card index systems 23, 24

Cases 13, 14
CD-ROM 14, 19
Cervical smears 6
CHD 21
Claims 1, 4, 5, 45, 140, 141
Clinical histories 3
Clinical records 23, 60
Coded items 10, 26, 71, 88
Coding systems 21, 26
Colour printers 19
Communications software 35, 148, 160
Complex searches 10, 49, 58, 63, 78, 90, 104
Consultation data 10, 55, 59, 80, 93, 105, 113, 119, 123, 128, 131
Contra-indications 73, 87, 112, 125
Convenience 3
Corel WordPerfect 54, 156, 157
CPUs 1, 13, 14, 17, 165
Cytology records 42

Data conversion charges 35
Data protection 35
Data handling 24, 53
Datafiles 162
Demonstrations 24, 25, 32–34, 38
Desktop 13, 113, 168
Diabetic templates 61, 74
Disease registers 3, 23, 60
Dispensing 30, 31, 92
Doctors' independent network 79
Dot matrix printers 18, 19

Drug recall 64
Dumb terminals 36, 113, 119, 123

EIDE 17
EISA 14, 165, 166
Electronic clinical records 60

Facilitation 37–38
FAR 75–76
Fileservers 14–16, 22, 36
Flat 26–27
Floppy disks 6, 17, 162, 169–172
FP10 18, 36, 46
Freehand screens 60, 61, 100
Frontdesk 89
Function keys 68–70, 73, 82, 113, 114, 117, 130

Generic forms 48, 87, 130
Gigabyte 16
GIGO 50

Hard disks 1, 6, 14, 16, 17, 36, 167–171
Health authorities 1, 5, 6, 24, 44, 139, 140
Health authority download 8, 35, 43–45
Health promotion 9, 25, 74
Helplines 8, 35, 148
Hierarchical 26, 27
High level code 26, 27
High speed serial ports 16, 168

176

Index

IBM compatibility 12, 166
IBM PCs 6
ICD9 27
ICD10 27
Indexes 3, 23, 24
Inkjet printers 18, 19, 159
Internet service providers 143, 147
I/O ports 16
IOS links 4, 67, 140, 141
ISA 14, 165, 166
ISDN 148

Keyboards 14, 17, 48, 124, 166

LANs 11, 13, 36, 67, 107, 128, 132, 165
Landlines 31, 32
Laser printers 18, 19, 159
Lloyd George 2, 23
Lotus 123 8, 152
LV1 92

Macros 48, 92, 100, 101, 105, 165, 170
Mailings 10, 25
Maintenance 8, 21–23
Major events 55, 59
Markers 134
Medical histories 59–60, 97–101, 104, 129, 130
Medical records 83–84, 88
Medication screens 69, 70, 72
Megabyte 1, 15, 16, 166
Memory 1, 14–17, 166
MENTOR 81
Merge 54, 55, 110, 122
Micros for GPs 6
Microsoft Excel 8, 66, 135, 152–156, 162, 174
Microsoft Word 54, 110, 135, 143, 156, 157, 162, 163, 170, 172
Mini towers 13
Modems 14, 16, 19, 31, 32, 92, 148, 149, 160, 165, 166
Monitors 13, 14, 17, 67, 81, 87, 167, 168, 170, 171
Motherboards 14–16
Mouse ports 16
MPRII standard 17
MS-DOS 18, 81, 132, 151, 156, 157, 161, 162, 166
Multi-user 11–13, 36, 67, 81, 119, 165, 166
Multiple disease registers 60
Multiplexers 11, 36, 67, 81, 95
MUMPS 18, 81, 166

National Coding Centre 29
Networks 11, 13, 16, 18, 35, 36, 67, 132, 145, 147, 165, 166, 171
Non-generic forms 48
Non-dispensing 31
Normal values 63
Notes screens 69–70, 72–75
Numeric data 58

Operating systems 18, 67, 81, 95, 119, 122, 151, 158, 161, 165, 166, 170
Opportunistic data entry 44, 56
OXMIS 27, 60, 95, 98, 99, 103, 105, 166

Paper records 23, 60
Paperless offices 7, 19, 23, 105, 136
Paperless practices 92, 93, 123
Parallel ports 16
Passwords 2, 59
PCG 1, 5
PCI 14, 165, 166
Pentium II 15, 16, 167
Pentium MMX 15, 168
Physical security 58, 59, 171
Pick 82
PILS 82
Practice Computing 30, 35, 173
Practice formularies 47, 48
Prescribing 46–48, 99
Private patients 54
Problem-oriented approaches 61, 71
Processors 14, 15, 165, 167, 168
Prodigy 81
Project managers 40, 41
Protocols 1, 6, 10, 11, 62, 63, 67, 73, 74, 79, 83, 88, 89, 116, 117
PULSE 30, 35

Quotations 32, 33

Radiation 17
RAM 1, 14–16, 107, 166–170
RCGP 27
Read codes 10, 21, 25–29
Registration 1, 5, 9, 10, 24, 35, 39, 41, 43–46, 49, 54, 68, 82, 96, 108, 114, 120, 123, 128, 133
Registration details 3, 164–166
Registration links 4, 9, 45, 54, 67, 96, 120, 139, 140
Registration status 45, 46, 54
Reminder letters 54
Repeat prescriptions 2, 4, 5, 9, 21–25, 29, 36, 40, 43, 46, 47, 61, 73, 99, 100, 110, 117, 124
Report generators 49,

76, 77, 79, 102–104, 128, 130–133, 136
Reports 63, 101, 103
Resolutions 17
RFA 7, 119
Road shows 24

Scanning 10, 19, 170
SCSI 17
Searches 22, 26, 46, 49, 51, 58, 64, 65, 89, 90, 92, 103, 104, 120, 122, 129, 139
Sequential data entry 44, 64
Shortlists 29, 38
Simple searches 9, 10, 39, 49, 63
Single page guides 47
SOPHIE 62, 67, 73–75, 79, 88, 89, 116, 117, 119, 166
Specifications 7, 13, 15, 17, 36, 38, 107, 167, 168
Spreadsheets 8, 22, 36, 66, 91, 112, 118, 143, 152–157, 160–163, 170, 172, 174
Standard reports 10, 50, 75, 89, 100–102, 122, 126

Stock control 31, 92
Structured records 60, 61, 86, 88, 95
Subcodes 26, 28, 71
Support maintenance 8, 22, 23, 35, 80, 93, 105, 113, 119, 123, 128, 131, 136
Support record 35
SVGA 17
Systems analysis 24

Target data 2
Targets 1, 24, 25, 49, 75, 126, 135
Telemedicine 6, 142, 144, 145
Templates 5, 10, 11, 31, 54, 61–63
Terminal emulation software 67, 81, 82, 92, 95, 119, 166
Torex 27, 107, 119, 123–128, 173
Training sessions 23, 40, 47

UNIX 18, 67, 113, 119, 123
Update 27
USB 16

User groups 62, 74
User interface 22, 29, 105, 165
User-defined reports 75, 126, 128

VAMP 7, 11, 27, 60–62, 81, 95–105, 107, 110–113, 118, 119, 121, 127, 129, 137, 165, 166, 173
Video cards 17, 166, 168
VL 14

Wide area networks 35
Windows 3.1 18
Windows 95/98 18, 92, 148, 151, 156, 168
Windows NT Server 81, 123, 148, 174
Word processing 8, 22, 82, 100, 110, 151, 152, 156, 160, 163, 170
Workstations 18, 107, 167, 168

XENIX 18, 67, 162
XGA 17, 168